Medical Abbreviations Pocket Guide

Copyright © 2022 Coventry House Publishing

All rights reserved.

ISBN: 1736696122
ISBN-13: 978-1736696125

Disclaimer

According to The Joint Commission, by using and promoting safe practices and by educating one another about hazards, medical professionals can better protect their patients. Therefore we recommend that you consult the following resources for a complete list of abbreviations and acronyms that have contradictory or ambiguous meanings before using this guide.

- Institute for Safe Medication Practices (www.ismp.org)
- ConsumerMedSafety (www.consumermedsafety.org)
- The Joint Commission (www.jointcommission.org)

These resources are updated regularly and often include a description of the potential problem along with the suggested correction. Abbreviations and acronyms currently appearing on the above referenced lists as of the date this book was published are marked with an asterisk (*) in the pages that follow.

A	ampere; angstrom
ā	before (ante)
A1c	glycated hemoglobin
A2	aortic second sound
AA	acetic acid; acute appendicitis; affected area; African American; Alcoholics Anonymous; alopecia areata; amino acid; aortic aneurysm; atlanto-axial
aa, āā	of each (ana ana)
A-a gradient	alveolar-arterial gradient
AAA	abdominal aortic aneurysm; apply to affected area
AAD	antibiotic-associated diarrhea
AAHPM	American Academy of Hospice and Palliative Medicine
AAI	acute arterial insufficiency
AAJ	atlanto-axial joint
AAL	anterior axillary line
AAMC	Association of American Medical Colleges
AAMI	age-associated memory impairment
AA&O, AAO	awake, alert, and oriented
AAP	American Academy of Pediatrics
AAPMC	antibiotic-associated pseudomembranous colitis
AAR	after action report; after action review
AAROM	active assisted range of motion
AAS	acute abdominal series
AAT	activity as tolerated; ambulate as tolerated; atypical antibody test
AAU	acute anterior uveitis

Ab	antibody
ab	abdomen/abdominal; abortion
A/B ratio	acid to base ratio
ABC	absolute basophil count; airway, breathing, circulation; aspiration biopsy cytology; automated blood count
ABCD	asymmetry, borders, color, diameter
ABCD^2	age, blood pressure, clinical findings, duration of symptoms, diabetes mellitus
ABCDE	airway, breathing, circulation, disability, exposure
abd	abdomen/abdominal; abduction
ABE	acute bacterial endocarditis
ABG	arterial blood gas
ABI	acquired brain injury; ankle-brachial index
ABLA	acute blood loss anemia
ABMT	autologous bone marrow transplant
abn	abnormal
ABO	blood group system
ABP*	acute bacterial prostatitis; ambulatory blood pressure*; arterial blood pressure*
ABPA	allergic bronchopulmonary aspergillosis
ABPI	ankle-brachial pressure index
ABR	auditory brain response
abs	absence; absent
ABW	actual body weight; adjusted body weight
ABX, ATB	antibiotic
AC	abdominal circumference; acromioclavicular; adrenal cortex; air conduction; antecubital; anterior chamber; anticoagulant; axiocervical

ac	before meals (ante cibos)
ac phos, ACP	acid phosphatase
ACA	Affordable Care Act; anterior cerebral artery; anticentromere antibody
ACB	aortocoronary bypass
ACC	acinic cell carcinoma; adenoid cystic carcinoma; ambulatory care center; aplasia cutis congenita
acc	accident; accommodation; according
accel	acceleration
ACCU	acute coronary care unit
ACD	allergic contact dermatitis; anemia of chronic disease; anticonvulsant drug
ACDF	anterior cervical discectomy and fusion
ACE	adverse clinical event; all-cotton elastic bandage; angiotensin-converting enzyme
ACEI	angiotensin-converting enzyme inhibitor
ACF	adult care facility
ACGME	Accreditation Council for Graduate Medical Education
ACh	acetylcholine
AChE	acetylcholinesterase
ACHES	abdominal pain, chest pain, headache, eye problems, severe leg pains
AChR	acetylcholine receptor
achs	before meals and at bedtime (ante cibos hora somni)
ACIP	Advisory Committee on Immunization Practices
ACL	anterior cruciate ligament
aCL	anticardiolipin antibody
ACLS	advanced cardiac life support

ACO	accountable care organization
ACOA	Adult Children of Alcoholics
ACOG	American Congress of Obstetricians and Gynecologists
ACP	acid phosphatase; advance care planning; advanced clinical practice
ACPO	acute colonic pseudo-obstruction
ACS	accountable care system; acute chest syndrome; acute coronary syndrome; ambulatory care sensitive; American Cancer Society
ACSC	ambulatory care sensitive conditions
ACT	activated clotting time; anticoagulant therapy
ACTH	adrenocorticotropic hormone
ACU*	acute receiving unit*; ambulatory care unit*
ACV	assist-control ventilation
ACVD	acute cardiovascular disease; atherosclerotic cardiovascular disease
AD*	acute distress; advance directive; Alzheimer's dementia; Alzheimer's disease; aortic dissection; atopic dermatitis; autosomal dominant; right ear (auris dextra)*
ad	up to
A&D	ascending and descending
ad lib	as desired (ad libitum)
ad part dolent	to the painful parts (ad partes dolentes)
ad sat	to saturation
ADA	adenosine deaminase; American Diabetes Association; American Dental Association; Americans with Disabilities Act
ADAP	AIDS Drug Assistance Program

ADC	AIDS-dementia complex; apparent diffusion coefficient
ADCC	antibody-dependent cellular cytotoxicity
ADD	attention deficit disorder
ADDH	attention deficit disorder with hyperactivity
addl	additional
ADE	adverse drug effect; adverse drug event; adverse drug experience
adeq	adequate
ADH	antidiuretic hormone
ADHC	Adult Day Health Care
ADHD	attention deficit hyperactivity disorder
ADHF	acute decompensated heart failure
ADHR	autosomal dominant hypophosphatemic rickets
ADI	acceptable daily intake
ADL	activity of daily living
adm	administer; admission; admit
ADME	absorption, distribution, metabolism, excretion
admin	administer; administration
admov	apply; let it be applied (admoveatur)
ADP	adenosine diphosphate
ADR	acute dystonic reaction; adverse drug reaction
ADT	admission, discharge, transfer; anticipated discharge tomorrow
ADTP	Alcohol and Drug Treatment Program
adv	advise
AE	above elbow; acute exacerbation; adverse event; arm ergometer
A&E	accident and emergency

AEA	above elbow amputation
AEB	as evidenced by
AEC	ambulatory emergency care
AED	antiepileptic drug; automated external defibrillator
AEE	activity energy expenditure
AEM	ambulatory event monitor
AER	adverse event report; auditory evoked response
aer	aerosol
AF	acid-fast; amniotic fluid; anteflexed; atrial fibrillation; atrial flutter
AFB	acid-fast bacillus; acid-fast bacteria
AFI	amniotic fluid index
A-fib, AF	atrial fibrillation
AFO	ankle-foot orthosis
AFP	alpha-fetoprotein
AFV	amniotic fluid volume
AFX	atypical fibroxanthoma
Ag	antigen; silver
A/G ratio	albumin to globulin ratio
AGA	anti-gliadin antibody; appropriate for gestational age; average for gestational age
AGC	atypical glandular cell
AGE	acute gastroenteritis
AGEP	acute generalized exanthematous pustulosis
AGES	age, grade, extent, size
agg, aggl	agglutination
agit	shake or stir (agita)
AGN	acute glomerulonephritis

AGNP	Adult-Gerontology Nurse Practitioner
AH	auditory hallucination
ah, alt hor	every other hour; alternate hours (alternis horis)
AHA	American Heart Association; American Hospital Association
AHC	acute hemorrhagic cystitis
AHCA	American Health Care Association
AHEC	Area Health Education Center
AHF	antihemophilic factor
AHG	aggregated human immunoglobulin G; antihemophilic globulin; antihuman globulin
AHH	aryl hydrocarbon hydroxylase
AHI	apnea-hypopnea index
AHIMA	American Health Information Management Association
AHIP	America's Health Insurance Plans
AHP	allied health professional
AHR	airway hyperresponsiveness
AHRQ	Agency for Healthcare Research and Quality
AI	adequate intake; aortic incompetence; aortic insufficiency; artificial insemination
AIAN	American Indian or Alaska Native
AICD	automatic implantable cardioverter defibrillator
AID	artificial insemination by donor
AIDP	acute inflammatory demyelinating polyneuropathy
AIDS	acquired immunodeficiency syndrome
AIH	artificial insemination, homologous; artificial insemination by husband; autoimmune hepatitis
AIHA	autoimmune hemolytic anemia

AIMS	Abnormal Involuntary Movement Scale; Arthritis Impact Measurement Scale
AIN	acute interstitial nephritis
AIP	acute interstitial pneumonia
AIPD	autoimmune progesterone dermatitis
AIR	anterior interval release
AIS	adenocarcinoma in situ; androgen insensitivity syndrome
AIVR	accelerated idioventricular rhythm
AJCC	American Joint Committee on Cancer
AK	above knee; Acanthamoeba keratitis; actinic keratosis
AKA	above knee amputation; also known as
AKI	acute kidney injury
AKN	acne keloidalis nuchae
ALA	aminolevulinic acid
alb	albumin
ALC	acute lethal catatonia; alternate level of care
alc	alcohol
ALCAPA	anomalous left coronary artery from the pulmonary artery
ALD	adrenoleukodystrophy; alcoholic liver disease
ALFT	abnormal liver function test
ALG	antilymphocyte globulin
ALI	acute limb ischemia; acute lung injury
alk	alkaline
ALL	acute lymphoblastic leukemia; acute lymphocytic leukemia
ALND	axillary lymph node dissection

ALOS	average length of stay
ALP, AP	alkaline phosphatase
ALPS	autoimmune lymphoproliferative syndrome
ALS	advanced life support; amyotrophic lateral sclerosis
ALT	alanine aminotransferase; alanine transaminase
alt	alternate/alternating; alternative
alt dieb	every other day (alternis diebus)
alt hor, ah	every other hour; alternate hours (alternis horis)
alt noc	every other night; alternate nights (alternis noctes)
AM, am	morning; before noon (ante meridiem)
AMA	advanced maternal age; against medical advice; antimitochondrial antibody; American Medical Association
amb	ambulate/ambulatory
AMC	academic medical center; arthrogryposis multiplex congenita
AMD	age-related macular degeneration; aging macular degeneration
AME	absorption, metabolism, excretion
AMI*	acute mesenteric ischemia; acute myocardial infarction*; anterior myocardial infarction*
AMIA	American Medical Informatics Association
AML	acute myeloid leukemia
AMLS	Advanced Medical Life Support
AMML	acute myelomonocytic leukemia
amnio	amniocentesis; amniotic
AMP	adenosine monophosphate
amp	ampere; ampule; amputate

AMR	antimicrobial resistance
AMS	acute mountain sickness; altered mental status; aseptic meningitis syndrome; atypical measles syndrome
AMSIT	appearance, mood, sensorium, intelligence, thought process
amt	amount
AMU	acute medical unit
AN	acanthosis nigricans
ANA	antinuclear antibody; antinuclear antigen
anast	anastomosis
anat	anatomic/anatomical; anatomy
ANC	absolute neutrophil count
ANCA	antineutrophilic cytoplasmic antibody
AND	allow natural death
ANDI	aberrations of normal development and involution
ANED	alive, no evidence of disease
anes, anesth	anesthesia
ANF	atrial natriuretic factor
ang, angio	angiogram; angiography
ANLL	acute nonlymphocytic leukemia
ANNA	anti-neuronal nuclear antibody
ANP	Adult Nurse Practitioner; Advanced Nurse Practitioner; atrial natriuretic peptide
ANS	autonomic nervous system
ant	anterior
ante	before
anti-CCP	anti-cyclic citrullinated peptide

anti-GBM	anti-glomerular basement membrane
ANUG	acute necrotizing ulcerative gingivitis
AO	atlanto-occipital
A&O	alert and oriented
A&Ox3	alert and oriented to person, place, and time
A&Ox4	alert and oriented to person, place, time, and situation
AOB	alcohol on breath
AODM	adult-onset diabetes mellitus
AOE	acute otitis externa
AOJ	atlanto-occipital joint
AOM	acute otitis media
AP	abdominal perineal; action potential; alkaline phosphatase; angina pectoris; antepartum; anterior-posterior; anteroposterior; apical pulse; area postrema
ap	before a meal (ante prandium)
A&P	anatomy and physiology; anterior and posterior; assessment and plan; auscultation and palpitation; auscultation and percussion
APA	anti-pernicious anemia; American Psychiatric Association
APACHE	Acute Physiology and Chronic Health Evaluation
APAP	N-acetyl-para-aminophenol (acetaminophen, paracetamol)
APC	activated protein C; admitted patient care; advanced patient care; advanced primary care; antigen-presenting cell; aspirin, phenacetin, caffeine; atrial premature contraction; argon plasma coagulation

APD	adult polycystic disease; afferent pupillary defect; anteroposterior diameter; automated peritoneal dialysis
APE	acute psychotic episode
APECED	autoimmune polyendocrinopathy-candidiasis-ectodermal dystrophy
APGAR	appearance, pulse, grimace, activity, respiration
APH	antepartum hemorrhage
API	active pharmaceutical ingredient
APKD	adult polycystic kidney disease
APL	antiphospholipid; abductor pollicis longus
APMPPE	acute posterior multifocal placoid pigment epitheliopathy
APMS	alternative provider medical services
APN	Advanced Practice Nurse
APORF	acute postoperative renal failure
appar	apparent
APPG	aqueous procaine penicillin G
applic	to be applied (applicandus)
approx	approximately
appt	appointment
appy	appendectomy
APR	abdominoperineal resection
APR-DRG	All Patient Refined Diagnosis Related Group
APRN	Advanced Practice Registered Nurse
APRV	airway pressure release ventilation
APS	Adult Protective Services; antiphospholipid syndrome; autoimmune polyglandular syndrome
APSAC	anisoylated plasminogen streptokinase activator complex

APSGN	acute poststreptococcal glomerulonephritis
APT	Anatomical Pathology Technologist
aPTT	activated partial thromboplastin time
aq, aqua	aqueous; water
aq ad	add water up to (aqua ad)
aq calid	warm water (aqua calida)
aq dest	distilled water (aqua destillata)
aq gel	cold water (aqua gelida)
AR	allergic rhinitis; aortic regurgitation; attributable risk; autosomal recessive
A-R	apical-radial
ARB	angiotensin receptor blocker
ARBD	alcohol-related birth defect; alcohol-related brain damage
ARBI	alcohol-related brain injury
ARC	acid-resistant cell; AIDS-related complex; American Red Cross
ARD	acute respiratory disease; alcohol-related dementia
ARDD	alcohol-related developmental disability
ARDS	acute respiratory distress syndrome; adult respiratory distress syndrome
ARF	acute renal failure; acute respiratory failure; acute rheumatic fever
ARM, AROM	artificial rupture of membranes
ARMD, AMD	age-related macular degeneration
ARMS	alveolar rhabdomyosarcoma
ARND	alcohol-related neurodevelopmental disorder
ARNP	Advanced Registered Nurse Practitioner

AROM	active range of motion; artificial rupture of membranes
ARRP	anatomic retropubic radical prostatectomy
ARRT	Adult Rapid Response Team
ARS	acute radiation syndrome; anti-rabies serum
ART	active resistance training; antiretroviral therapy; assisted reproductive technology; assisted reproductive therapy
art	artery/arterial
ARV	AIDS-related virus; antiretroviral
ARVC	arrhythmogenic right ventricular cardio-myopathy
ARVD	arrhythmogenic right ventricular dysplasia
AS*	ankylosing spondylitis; aortic stenosis; arteriosclerosis; atherosclerosis; left ear (auris sinistra)*
as tol	as tolerated
ASA	acetylsalicylic acid; American Society of Anesthesiologists
ASAP	as soon as possible
ASB	asymptomatic bacteriuria
ASC	altered state of consciousness; ambulatory surgery center; atypical squamous cells
asc	ascending
ASCA	anti-Saccharomyces cerevisiae antibody
ASCO	American Society of Clinical Oncology
ASCP	American Society of Clinical Pathologists
ASCUS	atypical squamous cells of undetermined significance
ASCVD	atherosclerotic cardiovascular disease

ASD	atrial septal defect; autism spectrum disorder
ASH	alcoholic steatohepatitis; asymmetric septal hypertrophy
AsH	hypermetropic astigmatism
ASHD	arteriosclerotic heart disease
ASHF	acute systolic heart failure
ASIS	anterior superior iliac spine
ASL	arterial spin labeling
ASLO, ASO	antistreptolysin O
AsM	myopic astigmatism
ASPECTS	Alberta Stroke Program Early CT Score
asst	assist/assistance
AST	aspartate aminotransferase
astigm, ast	astigmatism
ASU	acute surgical unit; ambulatory surgical unit
ASx	asymptomatic
AT	anterior tibial; antithrombin; atrial tachycardia
ATB, ABX	antibiotic
ATC	around-the-clock
ATCC	American Type Culture Collection
ATG	antithymocyte globulin
ATLS	advanced trauma life support
ATN	acute tubular necrosis
ATNR	asymmetrical tonic neck reflex
ATOD	alcohol, tobacco, other drugs
ATP	adenosine triphosphate; antitachycardia pacing; autoimmune thrombocytopenic purpura
atr	atrophy
ATR-BC	Registered Art Therapist-Board Certified

AU*	angstrom unit; arbitrary unit; both ears/each ear (auris uterque)*
AUC	area under the curve
aud	auditory
aug	augmentation
AUL	acute undifferentiated leukemia
AUS	artificial urinary sphincter
ausc, auscul	auscultation
aux	auxiliary
AV	actuarial value; anteverted; aortic valve; arteriovenous; atrioventricular
AVB	atrioventricular block
AVD	aortic valve disease; atrioventricular dissociation
AVF	arteriovenous fistula
AVG	Ambulatory Visit Group
avg	average
AVM	arteriovenous malformation
AVN	atrioventricular node; avascular necrosis
AVNRT	atrioventricular nodal reentrant tachycardia
$A\text{-}VO_2$	arteriovenous oxygen
AVP	arginine vasopressin
AVPU	alert, verbal, pain, unresponsive
AVR	aortic valve repair; aortic valve replacement
AVS	arteriovenous shunt
AVSD	atrioventricular septal defect
AVSS	afebrile, vital signs stable
AW, at wt	atomic weight
A&W	alive and well
a/w	admitted with; associated with

AWC	adequate and well-controlled
AWHONN	Association of Women's Health, Obstetric and Neonatal Nurses
AWMI	anterior wall myocardial infarction
ax	axillary
AXR	abdominal x-ray
AXT	alternating exotropia
AYA	adolescents and young adults
B	boron
Ba	barium
BAC	blood alcohol concentration; blood alcohol content; bronchoalveolar cell
bact	bacteria/bacterial
BAD, BPAD	bipolar affective disorder
BaE, BE	barium enema
BAEP	brainstem auditory evoked potential
BAER	brainstem auditory evoked response
BAHA	bone anchored hearing aid
BAL	blood alcohol level; bronchoalveolar lavage
bal	balance
BAO	basal acid output
barb	barbiturate
BASFI	Bath Ankylosing Spondylitis Functional Index
baso	basophil
BAT	brown adipose tissue
BAV	bicuspid aortic valve
BAVD	bicuspid aortic valve disease
BB	beta blocker; blood bank; breakthrough bleeding

BBA	bilateral breast augmentation
BBB	blood-brain barrier; bundle branch block
BBP	bloodborne pathogen
BBPS	Boston Bowel Preparation Scale
BBS	bilateral breath sound
BBT	basal body temperature
BBW	black box warning
BC	birth control; board certified; bone conduction; breast cancer
B&C	board and care
BCA	bichloroacetic acid
BCAA	branched-chain amino acid
BCBS	Blue Cross Blue Shield
BCC	basal cell carcinoma
BCCTP	Breast and Cervical Cancer Treatment Program
BCE	bone collagen equivalent
BCG	bacillus Calmette-Guérin (vaccine)
BCLS	basic cardiac life support
BCM	body cell mass
BCNSP	Board Certified Nutrition Support Pharmacist
BCOP	Board Certified Oncology Pharmacist
BCP	birth control pill; blood chemistry profile
BCPP	Board Certified Psychiatric Pharmacist
BCPS	Board Certified Pharmacotherapy Specialist
BCx	blood culture
BD	bipolar disorder; birth date; brain dead; Buerger's disease
BDD	body dysmorphic disorder
BDI	Beck Depression Inventory

BDR	background diabetic retinopathy
bds	two times a day (bis die sumendum)
BE	bacterial endocarditis; barium enema; base excess; below elbow
BEA	below elbow amputation
BEAM	brain electrical activity mapping
BEE	basal energy expenditure
beg	begin/beginning
BEQ	bioequivalence
BET	benign essential tremor
bet, btw	between
BF	breast fed/breast feeding
BFP	bundle-forming pilus
BFR	blood flow rate
BG	blood glucose
BGAT	blood glucose awareness training
BGL	blood glucose level
BGM	blood glucose monitoring
BH	behavioral health
BHP	Basic Health Program
BHS	behavioral health services; beta-hemolytic streptococcus
BHU	behavioral health unit
Bi	bismuth
BIB	brought in by
bib	drink (bibere)
BIBA	brought in by ambulance
bid	twice a day (bis in die)
BIDS	bedtime insulin and daytime sulfonylureas

BIH	benign intracranial hypertension; bilateral inguinal hernia; bilateral inguinal herniorrhaphy
bilat, bil, BL	bilateral
bili	bilirubin
bin	twice a night (bis in noctis)
BIOT, BTD	biotinidase deficiency
BiPAP	bilevel positive airway pressure
BIS	bispectral index
BiVAD	biventricular assist device
biw, tw	twice a week
BK	below knee; bradykinin
BKA	below knee amputation
BL	baseline; bilateral; bronchial lavage; Burkitt lymphoma
bld, bl	blood
BLE	bilateral lower extremity; both lower extremities
BLL	blood lead level
BLS	basic life support
BM	bone marrow; bowel movement; breast milk
BMA	bone marrow aspiration
BMB, BMBx	bone marrow biopsy
BMC	bone marrow cell; bone mineral content
BMD	Becker muscular dystrophy; bone mass density; bone mineral density
BME	biomedical engineering
BMI	body mass index
BMIC	breast milk iodine concentration
bmk	birthmark
BMP	basic metabolic panel

BMR	basal metabolic rate
BMS	bare-metal stent; bone marrow suppression
BMT	bone marrow transplant
BMx	bilateral mastectomy
BNO	bowel not open
BNP	brain natriuretic peptide
BO*	bowel obstruction*; bowel open*
b/o	because of
BOA	born out of asepsis
BOH	Board of Health
bol	pill (bolus)
BOLT	bilateral orthotopic lung transplant
BOM	bilateral otitis media
BOOP	bronchiolitis obliterans organizing pneumonia
bOPV	bivalent oral polio vaccine
BOS	base of support
BOT	base of tongue
bot	bottle; bottom
BP	blood pressure; British Pharmacopeia; bullous pemphigoid
BPAD, BAD	bipolar affective disorder
BPCA	Best Pharmaceuticals for Children Act
BPD	biparietal diameter; bipolar disorder; borderline personality disorder; bronchopulmonary dysplasia
BPd	blood pressure, diastolic
BPH	benign prostatic hyperplasia; benign prostatic hypertrophy
BPM	beats per minute

BPP	biophysical profile
BPPV	benign paroxysmal positional vertigo
BPRS	Brief Psychiatric Rating Scale
BPS	bilateral partial salpingectomy
BPs	blood pressure, systolic
BPSD	behavioral and psychological symptoms of dementia
BPV	benign positional vertigo
BR	bathroom; bed rest; bilirubin
BRA	bilateral renal agenesis
brady	bradycardia
BRAIDED	benefits, risks, alternatives, inquiries, decision, explanation, documentation
BRAO	branch retinal artery occlusion
BRAT	bananas, rice, applesauce, toast
BRATTY	bananas, rice, applesauce, toast, tea, yogurt
BRB	bright red blood
BRBPR	bright red blood per rectum
BRC	biomedical research center
BRCA	breast cancer gene
BRFSS	Behavioral Risk Factor Surveillance System
BRM	biologic response modifier
BROW	barley, rye, oats, wheat
BRP	bathroom privileges
BRTO	balloon-occluded retrograde transvenous obliteration
BRU	biomedical research unit
BRVO	branch retinal vein occlusion
BS	blood sugar; bowel sound; breath sound

b/s	bedside
BSA	body surface area; bovine serum albumin
BSB	breath sounds bilateral
BSC	bedside commode; biological safety cabinet
BSE	bovine spongiform encephalopathy; breast self-examination
BSF	basal skull fracture
BSI	bloodstream infection
BSL	biosafety level; blood sugar level
BSLE	bullous systemic lupus erythematosus
BSN	Bachelor of Science in Nursing; bowel sounds normal
BSO	bilateral salpingo-oophorectomy
BS&O	bilateral salpingectomy and oophorectomy
BSOM	bilateral serous otitis media
BSP	bromsulphthalein
BSS	balanced salt solution
BST	breast stimulation test
BSU	base service unit
BT*	bedtime*; bioterrorism; bleeding time; brachytherapy
Bt	Bacillus thuringiensis
BTB	breakthrough bleeding
BTBV	beat-to-beat variability
BTD, BIOT	biotinidase deficiency
BTE	behind-the-ear
BTFS	breast tumor frozen section
BTL	bilateral tubal ligation
BTP	bladder training program; breakthrough pain

BTT	blunt thoracic trauma; bridge to transplantation
btw, bet	between
BU	burn up
bucc	inside cheek (buccal)
BUE	bilateral upper extremity
BUM	backup method
BUN	blood urea nitrogen
BV	bacterial vaginosis; bone volume
BVM	bag valve mask
BVP	biventricular pacing
BVT	bilateral ventilation tube
BW	birth weight; blood work; body weight
BWS	battered woman syndrome
Bx	biopsy
C	Calorie (kilocalorie); carbon; Celsius
$\bar{c}$	with (cum)
C diff	Clostridium difficile
C1, C2, etc.	cervical vertebrae (first, second, etc.)
CA	cardiac arrest; cardiac arrhythmia; chronological age; coronary artery; cortical area
Ca	calcium
ca	cancer; carcinoma
C&A	conscious and alert
CAA	coronary artery aneurysm; crystalline amino acid
CAAHEP	Commission on Accreditation of Allied Health Education Programs
CAB	carotid artery bruit; chest compressions, airway, breathing

CABG	coronary artery bypass graft
CABS	coronary artery bypass surgery
CAC	Cardiac Advisory Committee; Certified Addiction Counselor
CACT	carnitine-acylcarnitine translocase
CAD	computer-aided detection; coronary artery disease
CADASIL	cerebral autosomal dominant arteriopathy with subcortical infarcts and leukoencephalopathy
CAE	complement activity enzyme
CAG	coronary angiogram; coronary angiography
CAGE	cut down, annoyed, guilty, eye-opener
CAH	chronic active hepatitis; congenital adrenal hyperplasia; critical access hospital
CAHPS	Consumer Assessment of Healthcare Providers and Systems
Cal, C, kcal	kilocalorie
cal, c	calorie
CALLA	common acute lymphocytic leukemia antigen
CAM	cell adhesion molecule; complementary and alternative medicine
cAMP	cyclic adenosine monophosphate
canc, Cx	cancel
CAO	conscious, alert, oriented
CAP	community-acquired pneumonia
CaP	cancer of the prostate
cap	capillary; capitation; capsule; let the patient take (capiat)
CAPD	central auditory processing disorder; continuous ambulatory peritoneal dialysis

CARES Act	Coronavirus Aid, Relief, and Economic Security Act
CARF	Commission on Accreditation of Rehabilitation Facilities
CARP	confluent and reticulated papillomatosis
CASAC	Credentialed Alcoholism and Substance Abuse Counselor
cat	cataract
CAT scan	computed axial tomography scan
CatG, CTG	cathepsin G
cath	catheter/catheterization
CAU	child and adolescent unit; clinical assessment unit
Cauc	Caucasian
CAUTI	catheter-associated urinary tract infection
cav	cavity
CAVP	continuous arterial venous pressure
CB	carotid bruit; cerebellum; chronic bronchitis
c/b	complicated by
CBA	cost-benefit analysis
CBC	complete blood count
CBD	cannabidiol; closed bag drainage; common bile duct
CBDS	common bile duct stone
CBE	charting by exception; clinical breast exam
CBF	cerebral blood flow
CBG	capillary blood gas; corticosteroid-binding globulin
CBI	continuous bladder irrigation
CBLL	capillary blood lead level

CBP	chronic bacterial prostatitis
CBR	complete bed rest
CBRNE	chemical, biological, radiological, nuclear, explosive materials
CBS	casual blood sugar; chronic brain syndrome
CBSC	cord blood stem cell
CBT	cognitive behavioral therapy
CC	care coordinator; chief complaint; complication or comorbidity; critical care
cc*	cubic centimeter*; with food (cum cibo)
C&C	confirmed and compatible
CCA	calcium channel antagonist; clear cell adenocarcinoma
cca	approximately (circa)
CCB	calcium channel blocker
CCC	central corneal clouding; chronic care clinic
CCCA	central centrifugal cicatricial alopecia
CCD	Continuity of Care Document
CCDA	Consolidated Clinical Document Architecture
CCE	clubbing, cyanosis, edema
CCF	congestive cardiac failure
CCH	care closer to home
CCIIO	Center for Consumer Information and Insurance Oversight
CCK	cholecystokinin
CCK-PZ	cholecystokinin-pancreozymin
CCMS	clean catch midstream
CCOC	clear cell odontogenic carcinoma
C-collar	cervical collar

CCOT	calcifying cystic odontogenic tumor
CCP	clinical care pathway; cyclic citrullinated peptide
CCPD	continuous cycling peritoneal dialysis
CCR	cardiocerebral resuscitation
CCRC	continuing care retirement community
CCT	Certified Cardiographic Technician
CCU	cardiac care unit; clean catch urine; coronary care unit; critical care unit
CCV	critical closing volume
CCW	counterclockwise
CD	cardiovascular disease; celiac disease; cesarean delivery; chemical dependency; cluster of differentiation; Crohn's disease; communicable disease; controlled delivery; controlled drug; curative dose; current diagnosis
CD4	helper T cells (cluster of differentiation 4)
CD8	cytotoxic T cells (cluster of differentiation 8)
CDA	Certified Dental Assistant
CDAC	Clinical Data Abstraction Center
CDAD	Clostridium difficile-associated diarrhea
C&DB	cough and deep breath
CDC	Centers for Disease Control and Prevention
CDE	Certified Diabetes Educator; complete dental evaluation
CDH	congenital dislocation of hip
CDHF	chronic diastolic heart failure
CDI	central diabetes insipidus; clean, dry, intact; Clostridium difficile infection
CDMI	Clinical Digital Maturity Index
CDMR	cesarean delivery on maternal request

cDNA	complementary DNA
CDP	cytosine diphosphate
CDR	cup-to-disk ratio; cutaneous drug reaction
CDRH	Center for Devices and Radiological Health
CDT	Certified Dental Technician
CDU	chemical dependency unit; clinical decision unit
CEA	carcinoembryonic antigen; cost-effectiveness analysis; carotid endarterectomy; cultured epithelial autografts
ceph	cephalic
cert	certificate; certified
CF	Christmas factor; cystic fibrosis
C/F	chills/fever
CFA	colonization factor antigen; complement fixation assay; complement fixing antibody
CFC	chlorofluorohydrocarbon
CFIDS	chronic fatigue immune dysfunction syndrome
CFR	case fatality rate; Child Fatality Review
CFS	chronic fatigue syndrome
CFT	complement fixation test
CFTR	cystic fibrosis transmembrane regulator
CFU	colony-forming unit
CG	chorionic gonadotropin
cg, cgm	centigram
CGD	chronic granulomatous disease
CGL	chronic granulocytic leukemia
CGM	continuous glucose monitoring
cGMP	cyclic guanosine monophosphate
CGN	chronic glomerulonephritis

cGy	centigray
CH	clinical hold; congenital hypothyroidism
ch	chest; child
CHA	Catholic Health Association
$CHADS_2$	congestive heart failure, hypertension, age, diabetes mellitus, prior stroke or transient ischemic attack
CHAMPVA	Civilian Health and Medical Program of the Veterans Administration
CHAP	Community Health Accreditation Program
CHB	complete heart block
CHC	combined hormonal contraceptive; community health center
CHD	chronic heart disease; congenital heart defect; congenital heart disease; congenital hip dislocation; coronary heart disease
ChE	cholinesterase
chem	chemical; chemistry
chemo, CTx	chemotherapy
CHF	chronic heart failure; congestive heart failure; continuous hemofiltration
chg	change
CHHA	Certified Home Health Agency; Certified Home Health Aide
CHI	closed head injury
CHIME	College of Healthcare Information Management Executives
CHIP	Children's Health Insurance Program
CHL	conductive hearing loss
CHNA	community health needs assessment

CHO, COH	carbohydrate
chol	cholesterol
choly	cholecystectomy
CHPX	chickenpox
chr	chronic
CHT	closed head trauma; congenital hypothyroidism
CI	cardiac index; cochlear implant; confidence interval; coronary insufficiency
Ci	curie
CIA	collagen-induced arthritis
CIBH	change in bowel habits
CIC	circulating immune complex; clean intermittent catheterization; crisis intervention center
CICC	centrally inserted central catheter
CICU	cardiac intensive care unit; coronary intensive care unit
CIDP	chronic inflammatory demyelinating polyneuropathy
cig	cigarette
CIMF	chronic idiopathic myelofibrosis
CIN	cervical intraepithelial neoplasia; contrast-induced nephropathy
CINV	chemotherapy-induced nausea and vomiting
CIP	clean in place
circ	circulation; circumcision; circumference
CIS	carcinoma in situ
CIVI	continuous intravenous infusion
CJD	Creutzfeldt-Jakob disease
CJR	Comprehensive Care for Joint Replacement

CK	creatine kinase
CKC	cold knife conization
CKD	chronic kidney disease
CK-MB	creatine kinase-myocardial band
CLABSI	central line-associated bloodstream infection
CLARE	contact lens-induced acute red eye
CLAS	culturally and linguistically appropriate services
CLD*	chronic liver disease*; chronic lung disease*
CLI	central line infection
clin	clinic/clinical
CLL	chronic lymphocytic leukemia
CLN	cervical lymph node; Clinical Lead Nurse; Clinical Liaison Nurse
CLND	central lymph node dissection; complete lymph node dissection
CLO	cleft lip only
CLOD	Clinical Lead for Organ Donation
CLP	cleft lip and/or palate
clr	clear
CLS	capillary leak syndrome
CM	cardiomegaly; cardiomyopathy; case manager
cm	centimeter; cream
cm^2	square centimeter
cm^3, cc	cubic centimeter
CMA	Certified Medical Assistant
CMC	carpometacarpal
CMCJ	carpometacarpal joint
CMD	cystic medial degeneration
CME	continuing medical education

CMG	cystometrogram; cystometrography
CMHC	community mental health center
CMIO	Chief Medical Information Officer
CML	chronic myelogenous leukemia; chronic myeloid leukemia
CMMI	Center for Medicare and Medicaid Innovation
CMML	chronic myelomonocytic leukemia
CMO	care management organization; Chief Medical Officer; comfort measures only
CMP	cardiomyopathy; competitive medical plan; comprehensive metabolic panel; cytidine monophosphate
CMR	cardiovascular magnetic resonance; Chief Medical Resident
CMS	Centers for Medicare and Medicaid Services; chronic mountain sickness; circulation, motion, sensation
cms	to be taken tomorrow morning (cras mane sumendus)
CMT	Certified Medication Technician; cervical motion tenderness; Charcot-Marie-Tooth (disease); continuing medication and treatment
CMTC	cutis marmorata telangiectatica congenita
CMV	cytomegalovirus; controlled mechanical ventilator
CN	cranial nerve
cn	tomorrow night (cras nocte)
CNA	Certified Nurse Aide; Certified Nursing Assistant
CNE	Certified Nurse Educator; chronic nervous exhaustion

CNH	central neurogenic hyperventilation; chondrodermatitis nodularis helicis
CNM	Certified Nurse-Midwife
CNMT	Certified Nuclear Medicine Technologist
CNNP	Certified Neonatal Nurse Practitioner
CNO	Chief Nursing Officer
CNP	Certified Nurse Practitioner
CNR	closed nasal reduction
CNS	central nervous system; Clinical Nurse Specialist; Crigler-Najjar syndrome
cns	to be taken tomorrow night (cras nocte sumendus)
CNSC	Certified Nutrition Support Clinician
CNV	choroidal neovascularization
CNVM	choroidal neovascular membrane
CO	carbon monoxide; cardiac output; Certified Orthotist
c/o	care of; complains of
CO_2	carbon dioxide
COA	Certified Ophthalmic Assistant
CoA	coarctation of the aorta
COAD	chronic obstructive airway disease
coag	coagulation
COB	close of business; coordination of benefits
COBRA	Consolidated Omnibus Budget Reconciliation Act
COC	cauterization of the cervix; certificate of coverage; combined oral contraceptive
cocci	coccidioidomycosis
COCP	combined oral contraceptive pill

COG	center of gravity
COGME	Council on Graduate Medical Education
COH	carbohydrate; controlled ovarian hyperstimulation
COLD	chronic obstructive lung disease
COM	chronic otitis media
comp	complication; compound
COMT	catechol-O-methyltransferase; Certified Ophthalmic Medical Technologist
conc	concentrated/concentration
cond	condition
cong	congenital; congested
conj	conjunctiva
CoNS	coagulase-negative staphylococci
cont	continue
contra	contraindication
contrx, CTX	contraction
CO-OP	Consumer Operated and Oriented Plan
COP	cryptogenic organizing pneumonia
CoP	conditions of participation
copay	copayment
COPD	chronic obstructive pulmonary disease
CoPS	coagulase-positive staphylococci
CORE	Coordinated Outbreak Response and Evaluation
corr	correct/correction
COT	Certified Ophthalmic Technician
COTA	Certified Occupational Therapy Assistant
COVID-19	coronavirus disease 2019
COWS	Clinical Opiate Withdrawal Scale

COX	cyclooxygenase
CP	cardiopulmonary; cerebral palsy; Certified Prosthetist; chest pain; cicatricial pemphigoid; cleft palate; clinical pregnancy; constrictive pericarditis
C&P	crowning and pushing
CPA	cardiopulmonary arrest; cerebellopontine angle; carotid phonoangiogram; carotid phonoangiography; costophrenic angle
CPAP	continuous positive airway pressure
CPC+	Comprehensive Primary Care Plus
CPCI	Comprehensive Primary Care Initiative
CPCR	cardiopulmonary cerebral resuscitation
CPD	cephalopelvic disproportion; chronic pulmonary disease; congenital polycystic disease
CPE	carbapenemase-producing Enterobacteriaceae; cardiogenic pulmonary edema; chronic pulmonary emphysema; Clostridium perfringens enterotoxin
CPEP	Comprehensive Psychiatric Emergency Program
CPG	clinical practice guideline
CPHQ	Certified Professional in Healthcare Quality
CPHSS	Cincinnati Prehospital Stroke Scale
CPhT	Certified Pharmacy Technician
CPK	creatine phosphokinase
CPM	care plan meeting; continuous passive mobilizer; continuous passive motion; counts per minute
CPMI	chronic and persistent mental illness
CPO	Certified Prosthetist and Orthotist; cleft palate only

CPP	cerebral perfusion pressure
CPPD	calcium pyrophosphate deposition; cyclic perimenstrual pain and discomfort
CPPV	continuous positive pressure ventilation
CPR	cardiopulmonary resuscitation
CPS	Child Protective Services
CPT	chest physiotherapy; Current Procedural Terminology
CPU	chest pain unit
cpy	copy
CQI	clinical quality indicator; continuous quality improvement
CR	capsule retention; complete remission; conditioned reflex; controlled release
Cr, creat	creatinine
CRA	Clinical Research Associate
CRAMS	circulation, respiration, abdomen, motor, speech
CRAO	central retinal artery occlusion
CRB	Change Review Board; Clinical Reference Board
CRC	Certified Rehabilitation Counselor; colorectal cancer
CrCl	creatinine clearance
CRD	chronic renal disease; chronic respiratory disease; circadian rhythm disorder
CRE	carbapenem-resistant Enterobacteriaceae
CREST	calcinosis, Raynaud phenomenon, esophageal dysmotility, sclerodactyly, telangiectasia
CRF	cardiac risk factors; chronic renal failure; corticotropin-releasing factor

CrGN	crescentic glomerulonephritis
CRH	corticotropin-releasing hormone
CRI	catheter-related infection; chronic renal insufficiency
CRIF	closed reduction and internal fixation
CRISPR	clustered regularly interspaced short palindromic repeats
crit, HCT	hematocrit
CRL	crown-rump length
crm, cr, cm	cream
CRNA	Certified Registered Nurse Anesthetist
cRNA	chromosomal RNA
CRNH	Certified Registered Nurse Hospice
CRNP	Certified Registered Nurse Practitioner
CRO	clinical research organization; contract research organization
CRP	C-reactive protein
CRPC	castrate-resistant prostate cancer
CRPS	complex regional pain syndrome
CRR	consult review request
CRRT	continuous renal replacement therapy
CRS	chronic rhinosinusitis; congenital rubella syndrome; cytoreductive surgery
CRSD	circadian rhythm sleep disorder
CRS-R	Conners' Rating Scales-Revised
CRT	capillary refill time; cardiac resynchronization therapy; cathode ray tube; central retinal thickness; Certified Respiratory Therapist; chemoradiotherapy
CRTT	Certified Respiratory Therapy Technician

CRU	coronary rehabilitation unit
CRVO	central retinal vein occlusion
cryo	cryoprecipitate; cryosurgery; cryotherapy
CS	cardiac sphincter; cardiogenic shock; cesarean section; chondroitin sulfate; clinically significant; close supervision; compartment syndrome; completed stroke
C&S	culture and sensitivity
CSA	Controlled Substances Act
C-section, CS	cesarean section
CSF	cerebrospinal fluid; colony-stimulating factor
CSH	combat support hospital
CSHF	chronic systolic heart failure
CSM	circulation, sensation, movement
CSME	clinically significant macular edema
CSO	Chief Scientific Officer
CSOM	chronic suppurative otitis media
CSP	central sterile processing
CSPC	community specialist palliative care
C-spine	cervical spine
CSR	central serous retinopathy; Cheyne-Stokes respiration; cumulative survival rate
CSS	Churg-Strauss syndrome
C-SSRS	Columbia-Suicide Severity Rating Scale
CST	Certified Surgical Technologist; contraction stress test
CSU	cardiac surgery unit; catheter specimen of urine
CSVD	cerebral small vessel disease

CT	cardiothoracic; cervicothoracic; completion thyroidectomy; computed tomography; chest tube; cytotechnology; Cytotechnologist
CT scan	computed tomography scan
CTA	clear to auscultation; computed tomography angiogram; computed tomography angiography
CTAB	clear to auscultation bilaterally
CTAP	computed tomography during arterial portography
CTB	cease to breathe; chronic tuberculosis
CTC	common toxicity criteria
CTCL	cutaneous T-cell lymphoma
CTD	connective tissue disease
CTE	chronic traumatic encephalopathy
CTEPH	chronic thromboembolic pulmonary hypertension
CTG, CatG	cathepsin G
CTLSO	cervical thoracic lumbar sacral orthosis
CTM	cricothyroid membrane
CTO	cervical thoracic orthosis; chronic total occlusion; clinical trial outline; community treatment order
CTP	Child-Turcotte-Pugh; color, temperature, pulse; cytidine triphosphate
CTPA	computed tomographic pulmonary angiogram; computed tomographic pulmonary angiography
CTR	carpal tunnel release
ctr	control
CTRS	Certified Therapeutic Recreation Specialist
CTS	carpal tunnel syndrome

CTX, contrx	contraction
CTx, chemo	chemotherapy
CTZ	chemoreceptor trigger zone
CU	case unknown
CUC	chronic ulcerative colitis
CUD	carnitine uptake defect
cur	current
CV	cardiovascular
CVA	cardiovascular accident; cerebrovascular accident; costovertebral angle
CVAD	central venous access device
CVAT	costovertebral angle tenderness
CVB	coxsackievirus B
CVC	central venous catheter; chronic venous congestion
CVD	cardiovascular disease; cerebrovascular disease
CVID	common variable immunodeficiency
CVL	central venous line
CVOU	cardiovascular outpatient unit
CVP	central venous pressure
CVRB	critical value read back
CVS	cardiovascular system; chorionic villus sampling; clean-voided specimen
CVT	cerebral venous thrombosis
CVVH	continuous venovenous hemofiltration
CW	clockwise
c/w	compared with; consistent with; continue with
CWD	canal wall down
CWP	coal workers' pneumoconiosis

CWR	canal wall reconstruction
CWU	canal wall up
Cx	cancel; cervix; circumflex; culture
CXR	chest x-ray
CY	calendar year
CYS	Children and Youth Services
cysto	cystoscopic; cystoscopy
D5NS	dextrose 5% in normal saline
D5W	dextrose 5% in water
DA	developmental age
Da	dalton
D&A	drugs and alcohol
DAEC	diffusely adherent Escherichia coli
DAF	decay-accelerating factor
DAI	diffuse axonal injury
DALY	disability-adjusted life year
DAP	data, assessment, plan
DAPE	data, assessment, plan, evaluation
DAPT	dual antiplatelet therapy
DAR	data, action, response
DARE	data, action, response, education
DARP	data, action, response, plan
DASE	Denver Articulation Screening Examination
DASH	Dietary Approaches to Stop Hypertension
DAT	diet as tolerated
dau	daughter
DAW	dispense as written
DAWN	Drug Abuse Warning Network
DB	direct bilirubin; double-blind

dB	decibel
DB&C	deep breathing and coughing
DBD	donation after brain death
DBE	double balloon enteroscopy
DBP	diastolic blood pressure
DBS	deep brain stimulation; dorsal blocking splint; dried blood spot
DBT	dialectal behavioral therapy
D&C	dilation and curettage
d/c*, DC*	discharge*; discontinue*
DCBE	double-contrast barium enema
DCC, DCCV	direct current cardioversion
DCD	donation after cardiac death
DCDA	dichorionic diamniotic
DCIS	ductal carcinoma in situ
DCM	dilated cardiomyopathy
DCP	dynamic compression plate
dcSSc	diffuse cutaneous systemic sclerosis
DCT	distal convoluted tubule
DD	delivery date; developmental disability; diastolic dysfunction; dry dressing
D&D	dehydration and diarrhea
DDD	defined daily dose; degenerative disk disease
DDH	developmental dysplasia of the hip
DDI	dressing dry and intact
dDNA	denatured DNA
DDS	Doctor of Dental Surgery
DDST	Denver Developmental Screening Test
DDx	differential diagnosis

D&E	dilation and evacuation
DEA	Drug Enforcement Administration
DECA	Devereux Early Childhood Assessment
dec'd	deceased
decel	deceleration
decr	decrease
decub	decubitus
def	deficiency
defib	defibrillation
deg	degree
dehy, DH	dehydration
del	deliver/delivery
dep	dependent
dept	department
deriv	derive/derivative
derm	dermatology; Dermatologist
DES	drug-eluting stent; dry eye syndrome
desc	descent/descending
det	let it be given (detur)
dev	develop
DEXA, DXA	dual energy x-ray absorptiometry
DF	dorsiflexion
DFA	direct fluorescent antibody
DFE	dilated fundus examination
DFR	dialysate flow rate
DFS	Doppler flow study
DFSP	dermatofibrosarcoma protuberans
DFV	Doppler flow velocimetry
DG	dorsal gluteal

dg, dgm	decigram
DH	dehydration; dermatitis herpetiformis; developmental history
DHEAS	dehydroepiandrosterone sulfate
DHF	decompensated heart failure
DHR	dihydrorhodamine
DHS	dynamic hip screw
DHT	dihydrotestosterone; Dobhoff tube
DI	detrusor instability; diabetes insipidus; disability insurance
diab	diabetes
diag, Dx	diagnosis
diam	diameter
DIB	difficulty in breathing
DIC	disseminated intravascular coagulation
DICOM	Digital Imaging and Communications in Medicine
DID	dissociative identity disorder
dieb alt	every other day (diebus alternis)
dieb tert	every third day (diebus tertius)
DIF	direct immunofluorescence
diff	differential
DIL	drug-induced lupus
dil	dilate/dilation; dilute/dilution
DILI	drug-induced liver injury
dim	dimension; diminish; half (dimidius)
DIP	desquamative interstitial pneumonia; distal interphalangeal
diph	diphtheria

DIPJ	distal interphalangeal joint
dir	direct; direction
DIRA	deficiency of interleukin-1-receptor antagonist
dis	disabled; discontinue; discussed; disease; dislocation
disc, d/c*, DC*	discontinue
DISCUS	Dyskinesia Identification System Condensed User Scale
DISH	diffuse idiopathic skeletal hyperostosis
disloc	dislocate
disp	dispense
diss	dissolve
dissem	disseminate
dist	distal; distribute
DIT	diet induced thermogenesis
DIU	death in utero
div	divide/division
DJD	degenerative joint disease
DKA	diabetic ketoacidosis
DL	direct laryngoscopy
dL	deciliter
DLB	dementia with Lewy bodies
DLCO	diffusing capacity of the lungs for carbon monoxide
DLE	discoid lupus erythematosus
DLI	donor lymphocyte infusion
DLP	dyslipoproteinemia
DLS	dynamic lumbar stabilization
DLSO	distal lateral subungual onychomycosis

DLVC	double lumen vascular catheter
DM	dermatomyositis; diabetes mellitus
DMAC	disseminated Mycobacterium avium complex
DMARD	disease-modifying antirheumatic drug
DMAT	Disaster Medical Assistance Team
DMD	Doctor of Medicine in Dentistry; Duchenne muscular dystrophy
DME	durable medical equipment
DMI	diabetic muscle infarction; diaphragmatic myocardial infarction
DMR	direct myocardial revascularization
DMSO	dimethyl sulfoxide
DMx	double mastectomy
DN	dibucaine number
DNA	deoxyribonucleic acid
DNACPR	do not attempt cardiopulmonary resuscitation
DNAR	do not attempt resuscitation
DNH	do not hospitalize
DNI	do not intubate
DNK	do not know
DNKA	did not keep appointment
DNP	Doctor of Nursing Practice
DNR*	did not respond*; do not resuscitate*
DNS	deviated nasal septum
DNT	did not test
DO	Doctor of Osteopathic Medicine; doctor's orders
D&O	diagnostic and observation
d/o	died of; disorder

DOA	date of admission; dead on arrival; drug of abuse; duration of action
DOB	date of birth
DOC	drug of choice
DOD	date of death
DOE	date of examination; design of experiment; dyspnea on exertion
DOH	Department of Health
DOI	date of injury
DOL	day of life
dom	dominant
DON	Director of Nursing
DOPT	directly observed preventive therapy
DOS	date of service; day of surgery
dos	dose/dosage
DOT	directly observed therapy
DOU	direct observation unit
DP	distal pulse; dorsalis pedis
DPA	dual-photon absorptiometry; dorsalis pedis artery
dPAP	diastolic pulmonary artery pressure
DPGN	diffuse proliferative glomerulonephritis
DPI	dry powder inhaler
DPL	diagnostic peritoneal lavage
DPLD	diffuse parenchymal lung disease
DPM	Doctor of Podiatric Medicine
DPN	diabetic peripheral neuropathy
DPOA	durable power of attorney
DPT	diphtheria, pertussis, tetanus (vaccine)

DQ	developmental quotient
DR	delayed release; delivery room; diabetic retinopathy; diagnostic radiography
Dr	doctor
dr	dram
DRE	digital rectal examination
DRESS	drug reaction with eosinophilia and systemic symptoms
DRF	drip rate factor
DRG	diagnosis-related group
DRI	daily reference intake; dietary reference intake
drng	drainage
DRPLA	dentatorubral-pallidoluysian atrophy
DS	diopters sphere; Down syndrome
DSA	digital subtraction angiogram; digital subtraction angiography; donor-specific antibody
DSB	drug-seeking behavior
DSD	dry sterile dressing
dsDNA	double-stranded DNA
DSM	Diagnostic and Statistical Manual of Mental Disorders
DSME	diabetes self-management education
DSPS	diagnostic, screening, preventive services
dsRNA	double-stranded RNA
DST	decision support tool; dexamethasone suppression test
DSW	Doctor of Social Work
DT	delirium tremens; diphtheria, tetanus (vaccine)
d/t	due to

DTA	descending thoracic aorta
DTAD	drain tube attachment device
DTH	delayed-type hypersensitivity
DTI	deep tissue injury
DTML	deep transverse metacarpal ligament
DTP, DTaP	diphtheria, tetanus, pertussis (vaccine)
DTR	Dietetic Technician, Registered; deep tendon reflex
DU	decubitus ulcer; diagnosis undetermined; duodenal ulcer
DUB	dysfunctional uterine bleeding
DUE	drug usage evaluation
DUI	driving under the influence
dup	duplicate/duplication
DUR	drug usage review; drug utilization review
dur dolor	while pain lasts (durante dolore)
DV	daily value; distance vision; double vision; domestic violence
D&V	diarrhea and vomiting
DVI	deep venous insufficiency
DVT	deep vein thrombosis
d/w	discussed with
DWI	driving while intoxicated
Dx, diag	diagnosis
DXA, DEXA	dual energy x-ray absorptiometry
DZ, dis	disease
E. coli	Escherichia coli
EA	epidural anesthesia
E&A	evaluate and advise

EAA	essential amino acid
EAB	elective abortion
EAC	erythema annulare centrifugum; external auditory canal
EAEC	enteroaggregative Escherichia coli
eAG	estimated average glucose
EAHF	eczema, asthma, hay fever
EAM	external auditory meatus
EAPG	Enhanced Ambulatory Patient Group
EAR	estimated average requirement
EB	epidermolysis bullosa
EBA	epidermolysis bullosa acquisita
EBB, EBBx	endobronchial biopsy
EBBS	equal bilateral breath sound
EBCT	electron beam computed tomography
EBF	exclusively breastfed
EBH, EBHC	evidence-based healthcare
EBL	estimated blood loss
EBLL	elevated blood lead level
EBM	evidence-based medicine; expressed breast milk
EBNA	Epstein-Barr nuclear antigen
EBRT	external beam radiation therapy
EBT	electron beam tomography; evidence-based treatment
EBV	Epstein-Barr virus
EC	emergency center; emergency contraception; emergency contact; energy conservation; eye contact; enteric coating
ECASA	enteric-coated acetylsalicylic acid

ECC	emergency cardiac care; endocervical curettage; extracorporeal circulation
ECCE	extracapsular cataract extraction
ECD	endocardial cushion defect
ECF	extended care facility; extracellular fluid
ECG, EKG	electrocardiogram; electrocardiography
ECHO	enteric cytopathic human orphan
echo	echocardiogram; echocardiography
ECL	electrochemiluminescence
ECLAM	European Consensus Lupus Activity Measure
ECLS	extracorporeal life support
ECM	extracellular matrix
ECMO	extracorporeal membrane oxygenation
ECP	Emergency Care Practitioner; emergency contraceptive pill
eCQM	electronic clinical quality measure
ECR	emergency chemical restraint
ECRB	extensor carpi radialis brevis
ECRL	extensor carpi radialis longus
ECT	electroconvulsive therapy
ECU	emergency care unit; extended care unit; extensor carpi ulnaris
ECV	external cephalic version; extracellular volume
ED*	ectodermal dysplasia; effective dose; emotional disorder*; erectile dysfunction*
EDB	extensor digitorum brevis
EDC	estimated date of conception; estimated date of confinement; extensor digitorum communis
ED&C	electrodessication and curettage

EDD	end-diastolic diameter; estimated delivery date; estimated discharge date
EDF	end-diastolic flow
EDH	epidural hematoma
EDL	extensor digitorum longus
EDM	esophageal Doppler monitor
EDP	end-diastolic pressure; erythema dyschromicum perstans
EDR	electrodermal response
EDRF	endothelium-derived relaxing factor
EDS	Ehlers-Danlos syndrome
EDTA	ethylenediaminetetraacetic acid
edu	education
EDV	end-diastolic volume; epidermodysplasia verruciformis
EDX	electrodiagnostic
E&E	eye and ear
EED	erythema elevatum diutinum
EEE	eastern equine encephalitis
EEG	electroencephalogram; electroencephalography
EENT	eye, ear, nose, throat
EER	estimated energy requirement
EF	ejection fraction; eosinophilic fasciitis
EFAD	essential fatty acid deficiency
eff	effect/effective
EFM	electronic fetal monitoring
EFS	event-free survival
EFW	estimated fetal weight
EGA	estimated gestational age

EGBUS	external genitalia, Bartholin's glands, urethra and Skene's glands
EGC	early gastric cancer
EGD	esophagogastroduodenoscopic; esophagogastroduodenoscopy
EGF	epidermal growth factor
EGFR	epidermal growth factor receptor
eGFR	estimated glomerular filtration rate
EGG	electrogastrogram; electrogastrography
EGPA	eosinophilic granulomatosis with polyangiitis
EHB	essential health benefit; extended health benefit; extensor hallucis brevis
EHC	emergency hormonal contraception; eye-hand coordination
EHEC	enterohemorrhagic Escherichia coli
EHL	electrohydraulic lithotripsy; extensor hallucis longus
EHR	electronic health record
EHS	employee health service
EI	early intervention; endotracheal intubation
EIA	enzyme immunoassay; exercise-induced asthma; external iliac artery
EIB	exercise-induced bronchospasm
EIC	epidermal inclusion cyst
EID	early infant diagnosis; electronic infusion device
EIEC	enteroinvasive Escherichia coli
EIP	extensor indicis proprius
EIPV	enhanced-potency inactivated poliovirus vaccine
EIU	enzyme immunoassay unit

EJ	elbow jerk; external jugular
EKG, ECG	electrocardiogram; electrocardiography
el	elect/elective; elixir
elb	elbow
ELDU	extra-label drug use
elev	elevated
ELF	elective low forceps
ELISA	enzyme-linked immunosorbent assay
elix, el	elixir
ELS	endolymphatic shunt
EM	electron microscopy; emergency medicine; erythema multiforme
E&M	evaluation and management
eMAR	electronic Medication Administration Record
EMB, EMBx	endometrial biopsy; endomyocardial biopsy
emb	embryo
EMC	encephalomyocarditis; electromagnetic compatibility
EMCV	encephalomyocarditis virus
EMD	electromechanical dissociation
emer	emergency
EMF	endomyocardial fibrosis
EMG	electromyogram; electromyography
emot	emotion/emotional
emp	as directed (ex modo prescripto)
EMR	electronic medical record
EMS	electrical muscle stimulation; electrical muscle stimulator; emergency medical service; emergency medical system

EMT	Emergency Medical Technician
EMTALA	Emergency Medical Treatment and Labor Act
EMU	early morning urine
emuls	emulsion
EMV	eye, motor, verbal
EN	enteral nutrition; erythema nodosum
ENA	extractable nuclear antigen
endo	endocrine; endocrinology; Endocrinologist; endoscopic; endoscopy
ENE	extranodal extension
ENG	electronystagmogram; electronystagmography
ENL	erythema nodosum leprosum
enl	enlarged
ENT	ear, nose, throat
e/o	evidence of
EOA	esophageal obturator airway
EOB	edge of bed; explanation of benefits
EOD	end of day; every other day
EoE	eosinophilic esophagitis
EOG	electrooculogram; electrooculography
EOLC	end-of-life care
EOM	extraocular movement; extraocular muscles
EOMI	extraocular movement intact; extraocular muscle intact
EOP	Emergency Operation Plan
EOS	end of study
eos	eosinophil
EP	ectopic pregnancy; electrophysiology; extrapyramidal

EPB	extensor pollicis brevis
EPCT	estrogen-progesterone challenge test
EPEC	enteropathogenic Escherichia coli
EPEP	end positive expiratory pressure
EPH	edema, proteinuria, hypertension
epi	epidural; epinephrine
epis	episiotomy
epith	epithelial
EPL	extensor pollicis longus
EPO	erythropoietin; exclusive provider organization
EPR	electronic patient record; emergency physical restraint
EPS	elastosis perforans serpiginosa; extrapyramidal symptoms; electrophysiologic study
EPSDT	Early and Periodic Screening, Diagnostic, and Treatment
EPSE	extrapyramidal side effect
eq	equal
equip	equipment
equiv	equivalent
ER	emergency room; extended release; external rotation
ERCP	endoscopic retrograde cholangiopancreatography
ERG	electroretinogram; electroretinography
ERM	epiretinal membrane
ERMS	embryonal rhabdomyosarcoma
ERP	Emergency Response Plan
ERS	extended, rotated, side bent

ERT*	Emergency Resuscitation Team; enzyme replacement therapy*; estrogen replacement therapy*
ERV	expiratory reserve volume
ES	effect size; electrical stimulation; epidural steroid; extra strength
ESA	erythropoiesis-stimulating agent
ESBL	extended-spectrum beta-lactamase
ESD	end-systolic diameter; end-systolic dimension
eSET	elective single embryo transfer
ESG	estrogen signaling
ESI	employer-sponsored insurance; epidural steroid injection
eSig	electronic signature
ESLD*	end-stage liver disease*; end-stage lung disease*
ESM	ejection systolic murmur
ESR	erythrocyte sedimentation rate
ESRD	end-stage renal disease
ESRF	end-stage renal failure
ESS	empty sella syndrome
EST	electroshock therapy; endodermal sinus tumor
est	estimate
ESV	end-systolic volume
ESWL	extracorporeal shock wave lithotripsy
ET	embryo transfer; endotracheal; enterostomal therapy; Enterostomal Therapist; esotropia; essential thrombocythemia; estrogen therapy; eustachian tube
et	and

ETA	estimated time of arrival
ETCO$_2$	end-tidal carbon dioxide
ETD	eustachian tube dysfunction
ETEC	enterotoxigenic Escherichia coli
ETOH	ethanol; ethyl alcohol
ETP	elective termination of pregnancy
ETS	endoscopic thoracic sympathectomy; environmental tobacco smoke
ETT	endotracheal tube; exercise tolerance test; exercise treadmill test
ETU	emergency trauma unit; emergency treatment unit
EU	endotoxin unit; ELISA (enzyme-linked immunosorbent assay) unit
EUA	emergency use authorization; examination under anesthesia
EUP	extrauterine pregnancy
EUS	endoscopic ultrasound
EV	ELISA (enzyme-linked immunosorbent assay) value
evac	evacuate/evacuation
eval	evaluate/evaluation
EVAR	endovascular aneurysm repair
EVD	external ventricular drain
EVF	erythrocyte volume fraction
EVH	endoscopic vein harvesting
EWCL	extended wear contact lens
exam, ex	examination
exer	exercise
exp, expir	expire/expiration

expl	exploratory
ext	extend; extension; extensor; exterior; external; extract; extremity
F	Fahrenheit
FA	Fanconi anemia; fatty acid; femoral artery; folic acid; forearm; Friedreich's ataxia
FACS	Fellow, American College of Surgeons; fluorescence-activated cell sorter
FADL	functional activity of daily living
FAH	Federation of American Hospitals
FAI	free androgen index; Functional Assessment Inventory
FAM	fertility awareness method
fam, fm	family
FAMMM	familial atypical multiple mole melanoma
FANA	fluorescent antinuclear antibody
FAP	familial adenomatous polyposis
FAS	fetal alcohol syndrome
FAST	focused assessment with sonography for trauma
fax	facsimile
FB	fingerbreadth; foreign body
f/b	followed by
FBC	family birth center; full blood count
FBD, FCBD	fibrocystic breast disease
FBE	full blood examination
FBG	fasting blood glucose
FBM	fetal breathing movement
FBP	fetal biophysical profile
FBS	fasting blood sugar

FBSS	failed back surgery syndrome
F&C	fever and chills; foam and condoms
F/C	fever/chills
FCAS	familial cold autoinflammatory syndrome
FCBD, FBD	fibrocystic breast disease
FCE	functional capacity evaluation
FCHCO	Federal Coordinated Health Care Office
FCR	flexor carpi radialis
FCS	familial chylomicronemia syndrome
FCU	flexor carpi ulnaris
FD	fatal dose; focal distance; fully dilated
FDA	Food and Drug Administration
FDB	flexor digitorum brevis
FDC	fixed-dose combination; follicular dendritic cell
FDIU	fetal death in utero
FDL	flexor digitorum longus
FDLMP	first day of last menstrual period
FDP	fibrin degradation product; flexor digitorum profundus
FDS	flexor digitorum superficialis
Fe	iron
F&E	fluid and electrolytes
FEES	flexible endoscopic evaluation of swallowing
FEF	forced expiratory flow
FEHB	Federal Employees Health Benefits
fem	female; femoral
fem-pop, FP	femoropopliteal
FEN	fluids, electrolytes, nutrition
FENa	fractional excretion of sodium

FEP	fibroepithelial polyp; free erythrocyte protoporphyrin
FES	functional electrical stimulation
FESS	functional endoscopic sinus surgery
FET	forced expiratory technique; frozen embryo transfer
FEV	forced expiratory volume
FEV_1	forced expiratory volume in 1 second
FF	force fluids; free fluid; fundus firm
FFA	free fatty acid; frontal fibrosing alopecia
FFE	Federally Facilitated Exchange
FFF	fully formula fed
FFL	flexible fiberoptic laryngoscopy
FFM	Federally Facilitated Marketplace
FFP	fresh frozen plasma
FFPE	formalin-fixed paraffin-embedded
FFS	fee-for-service
FGT	female genital tract
FH, FHx	family history
FHB	flexor hallucis brevis
FHC	family health center
FHL	flexor hallucis longus
FHM	fetal heart monitoring
FHR	fetal heart rate
FHS	fetal heart sound
FHT	fetal heart tone
FI	fusion inhibitor
fib	fibrillation
FIH	first-in-human

FIM	Functional Independence Measure
FiO$_2$	fraction of inspired oxygen
FISH	fluorescence in situ hybridization
FL	femur length
fL	femtoliter
fl, fld	fluid
FLAIR	fluid-attenuated inversion recovery
flex	flexible; flexion
FLP	fasting lipid panel
flu	influenza
fluoro	fluoroscopic; fluoroscopy
FM	family medicine; fetal movement; fibromyalgia
fm, fam	family
FMC	family maternity center
FMD	fibromuscular dysplasia
FMF	fetal movement felt
FMG	Foreign Medical Graduate
FMP	first menstrual period
FMPP	familial male-limited precocious puberty
fMRI	functional magnetic resonance imaging
FMS	fibromyalgia syndrome; full mouth series
FMTE	full mouth tooth extraction
FN	febrile neutropenia
F&N	fever and neutropenia
FNA	fine needle aspiration
FNAB	fine needle aspiration biopsy
FNAC	fine needle aspiration cytology
FND	functional neurologic disorder
FNE	fiberoptic nasal endoscopy

FNH	focal nodular hyperplasia
FNP	Family Nurse Practitioner
FOB	father of baby; fiberoptic bronchoscopy; foot of bed
FOBT	fecal occult blood test
FOC	fronto-occipital circumference
FOD	free of disease
FOI	flight of ideas
FOM	floor of mouth
FOOSH	fall onto outstretched hand
FOP	fibrodysplasia ossificans progressiva
FOS	force of stream; full of stool
FP	Family Physician; family planning; family practice; Family Practitioner; femoropopliteal
FPCG	fetal phonocardiogram; fetal phonocardiography
FPEM	family planning education materials
FPG	fasting plasma glucose
FPIA	fluorescence polarization immunoassay
FPL	flexor pollicis longus
FQHC	Federally Qualified Health Center
FR	friction rub
frag	fragment
FRC	functional residual capacity
FRDA, FA	Friedreich's ataxia
freq	frequency
FRG	functional related group
FRJM	full range of joint movement
FROM	free range of motion; full range of motion

FRS	flexed, rotated, side bent
FRT	female reproductive tract
fru	fructose
FRV	functional residual volume
FRX, Fx, frac	fracture
FS	Felty's syndrome; finger stick; frozen section
FSA	flexible spending account
FSBG	finger stick blood glucose
FSBS	finger stick blood sugar
FSE	fetal scalp electrode
FSG	finger stick glucose
FSGS	focal segmental glomerulosclerosis
FSH	follicle-stimulating hormone
FSMB	Federation of State Medical Boards
FT	fingertip; full term; full time
ft	foot/feet
FTA	fluorescent treponemal antigen
FTD	frontotemporal dementia
FTI	free testosterone index
FTND	full-term normal delivery
FTP	failure to progress
FTSG	full-thickness skin graft
FTT	failure to thrive
f/u, FU	follow up
FUE	follicular unit extraction
func	function
FUO	fever of unknown origin
FUS	focused ultrasound surgery
FUT	follicular unit transplantation

FVC	forced vital capacity
FVD	fluid volume deficit
FVE	fluid volume excess
FWB	fetal wellbeing; follicle wall biopsy; full weight bearing
Fx, FRX, frac	fracture
FXD, x10d	for 10 days
FY	fiscal year
FYI	for your information
g, gm	gram
G-, GN	gram negative
G+, GP	gram positive
GA	general anesthesia; gestational age; granuloma annulare
G&A	general and acute
GABA	gamma-aminobutyric acid
GABHS	group A beta-hemolytic streptococcus
GAD	generalized anxiety disorder
GAF	Global Assessment of Functioning
GAG	glycosaminoglycan
gal	gallon
GALT	galactose-1-phosphate uridyltransferase
GAPS	Guidelines for Adolescent Preventative Services
garg	gargle
GAS	group A streptococcus; general adaptation syndrome
GAVE	gastric antral vascular ectasia
GB	gallbladder; Guillain-Barré
GBC	gallbladder carcinoma

GBM	glioblastoma multiforme; glomerular basement membrane
GBS	gallbladder series; group B streptococcus; Guillain-Barré syndrome
GC	glucocorticoid; gonococcus; gonorrhea
GCA	giant cell arteritis
GCS	Glasgow Coma Scale; graduated compression stocking; group C streptococcus
G-CSF	granulocyte-colony stimulating factor
GCT	germ cell tumor; giant cell tumor; glucose challenge test
GD	gender dysphoria
G&D	growth and development
GDA	gastroduodenal artery
GDH, GLDH	glutamate dehydrogenase
GDM	gestational diabetes mellitus
GDMT	guideline-directed medical therapy
GDP	guanosine diphosphate
GDS	group D streptococcus; Geriatric Depression Scale
GE	gastroenteritis; gastroesophageal
GEA, GETA	general endotracheal anesthesia
gen	general
GER	gastroesophageal reflux
ger	geriatric
GERD	gastroesophageal reflux disease
gest	gestation/gestational
GET	general endotracheal
GETT	general by endotracheal tube

GF	glomerular filtrate
GFM	good fetal movement
GFR	glomerular filtration rate
GG	gamma globulin
GGT	gamma-glutamyl transferase
GGTP	gamma-glutamyl transpeptidase
GH	glenohumeral; good health; growth hormone
GHB	gamma hydroxybutyrate
GHIF	growth hormone-inhibiting factor
GHIH	growth hormone-inhibiting hormone
GHRF	growth hormone-releasing factor
GHRH	growth hormone-releasing hormone
GI	gastrointestinal; glycemic index
GIB	gastrointestinal bleeding
GIFT	gamete intrafallopian transfer
GIST	gastrointestinal stromal tumor
GIT	gastrointestinal tract
GITS	gastrointestinal therapeutic system
gl	gland
GLP	Good Laboratory Practice
GLT	glucose loading test
glu, glc	glucose
glut	gluteal
GM	genetically modified
gm, g	gram
GMC	general medical condition
GM-CSF	granulocyte-macrophage colony-stimulating factor
GME	Graduate Medical Education

GMO	genetically modified organism
GMP	guanosine monophosphate
GMR	gallops, murmurs, rubs
GN	glomerulonephritis; Graduate Nurse; gram negative
GNA	Geriatric Nursing Assistant
GNB	gram-negative bacillus
GNC	gram-negative cocci
GNR	gram-negative rod
GnRH	gonadotropin-releasing hormone
GOAT	Galveston Orientation and Amnesia Test
GOC	goal of care
GOMER	"Get out of my emergency room!"
GOO	gastric outlet obstruction
GORD	gastro-oesophageal reflux disease
GOT	glutamic oxaloacetic transaminase
GOx	glucose oxidase
GP	general paralysis; general practitioner; general precaution; glycoprotein; gram positive
GPA	granulomatosis with polyangiitis
GPB	gram-positive bacillus
GPC	gram-positive cocci
GPN	glossopharyngeal neuralgia; Graduate Practical Nurse
GPR	gram-positive rod
GPS	Goodpasture syndrome
GPT	glutamic pyruvic transaminase
GR	grand rounds
gr	grain

grad	gradual
GRAS	generally recognized as safe
GRASE	generally recognized as safe and effective
grav	pregnancy (gravid)
grp	group
GRS	gender reassignment surgery
GS	general surgery; gram stain
GSW	gunshot wound
GT, G-tube	gastrostomy tube
GTCS	generalized tonic-clonic seizure
GTN	gestational trophoblastic neoplasia
GTT	gestational trophoblastic tumor; glucose tolerance test
gtt	drop (gutta)
gtts	drops (guttae)
GU	genitourinary; gonococcal urethritis; gastric ulcer
GUM	genitourinary medicine
guttat	drop by drop (guttatim)
GvHD	graft-versus-host disease
GvL	graft-versus-leukemia
GWG	gestational weight gain
GXT	graded exercise test
Gy	gray (unit)
gyn	gynecology; Gynecologist
H flu	Haemophilus influenzae
H1N1	hemagglutinin type 1 and neuraminidase type 1
H2	histamine-2
H_2O	water

HA	headache; Health Authority; hearing aid; hemolytic anemia
HAA	hepatitis-associated antigen
HAART	highly active antiretroviral therapy
HAC	healthcare-acquired condition; hospital-acquired condition
HACA	human anti-chimeric antibody
HACE	high-altitude cerebral edema
HAD	HIV-associated dementia
HADS	Hospital Anxiety and Depression Scale
HAE	hearing aid evaluation; hereditary angioedema
HAI	healthcare-acquired infection; hospital-acquired infection
HAIR-AN	hyperandrogenism, insulin resistance, acanthosis nigricans
HAL	hyperalimentation
HALE	health-adjusted life expectancy
HAM-D, HRSD	Hamilton Rating Scale for Depression
HAPE	high-altitude pulmonary edema
HAQ	Health Assessment Questionnaire
HARP	Health and Recovery Plan
HARRI	Home Assessment Resource Review Instrument
HART	High Acuity Response Team
HAV	hepatitis A virus
HAZMAT	hazardous material
HAZOP	hazard and operability
HB	heart block
Hb, Hgb, hem	hemoglobin
HbA, HbB, etc.	hemoglobin A, hemoglobin B, etc.

HbAS	hemoglobin A and hemoglobin S (sickle cell trait)
HbA1c	glycosylated hemoglobin
HBGM	home blood glucose monitoring
HBO	hyperbaric oxygenation
HBOT	hyperbaric oxygen therapy
HBP	high blood pressure
HBV	hepatitis B virus
HBW	horizontal bitewing
HC	head circumference; hemorrhagic colitis; home care; homocysteine; hydrocortisone
HCA	Health Care Aide; Health Care Assistant
HCAHPS	Hospital Consumer Assessment of Healthcare Providers and Systems
HCAP	healthcare-associated pneumonia
HCBS	home and community-based services
HCC*	hepatocellular carcinoma*; Hürthle cell carcinoma*
HCEARA	Health Care and Education Affordability Reconciliation Act
HCFA	Health Care Financing Administration
hCG	human chorionic gonadotropin
HCL	hairy cell leukemia; hard contact lens
HCl*	hydrochloric acid*; hydrochloride*
HCM	hypertrophic cardiomyopathy
HCO	health care organization
HCP	health care professional; health care provider
HCPCS	Healthcare Common Procedure Coding System
HCR	Health Care Reform
hCS	human chorionic somatomammotropin

HCT*	hematocrit; hematopoietic cell transplantation; hydrocortisone*
HCUP	Healthcare Cost and Utilization Project
HCV	hepatitis C virus
HCVD	hypertensive cardiovascular disease
HCW	healthcare worker
HCY, HCU	homocystinuria
Hcy	homocysteine
HD*	Hansen's disease*; Hodgkin's disease*; Huntington's disease*; health department; hearing distance; hemodialysis; herniated disk
hd, hor decub	at bedtime (hora decubitus)
HDC	high-dose chemotherapy
HDCV	human diploid cell vaccine
HDHP	high-deductible health plan
HDL	high-density lipoprotein
HDN	hemolytic disease of the newborn
HDRS	Hamilton Depression Rating Scale
HDS	hemodynamically stable
HDU	hemodialysis unit; high-dependency unit
HDV	hepatitis D virus
HDW	hemoglobin distribution width
HE	hepatic encephalopathy
H&E	hematoxylin and eosin
HEC	highly emetogenic chemotherapy
HEDIS	Health Employer Data and Information Set
HEENT	head, eyes, ears, nose, throat
HELLP	hemolysis, elevated liver enzymes, low platelets
hem	hematology; Hematologist; hemoglobin

hemi	half
HEP	home exercise program
HEPA	high-efficiency particulate air
HER2	human epidermal growth factor receptor 2
HERDS	Hospital Emergency Response Data System
HETE	hydroxyeicosatetraenoic acid
HEV	hepatitis E virus
HF	heart failure; high frequency
HFA	hydrofluoroalkane
HFCS	high-fructose corn syrup
HFMA	Healthcare Financial Management Association
HFMD	hand, foot, and mouth disease
HFNC	high-flow nasal cannula
HFpEF	heart failure with preserved ejection fraction
HFrEF	heart failure with reduced ejection fraction
HFRS	hemorrhagic fever with renal syndrome
HFV	hepatitis F virus
Hg	mercury
Hgb, Hb, hem	hemoglobin
HGF	hepatocyte growth factor; human growth factor
HGH	human growth hormone
HGSIL, HSIL	high-grade squamous intraepithelial lesion
hgt, ht	height
HGV	hepatitis G virus
HH	hiatal hernia
H&H	hemoglobin and hematocrit
HHA	home health agency; Home Health Aide
HHC	home health care
HHD	hypertensive heart disease

HHE	Health Hazard Evaluation
HHI	Herth Hope Index
HHN	handheld nebulizer
HHQI	Home Health Quality Initiative
HHRG	Home Health Resource Group
HHS	Department of Health and Human Services; hyperosmolar hyperglycemic syndrome
HHT	hereditary hemorrhagic telangiectasia
HHV	human herpesvirus
HI	health insurance; hemagglutination inhibition; hepatic insufficiency; homicidal ideation
HIA	Health Impact Assessment
HIAA	Health Insurance Association of America
Hib	Haemophilus influenzae type B
HID	herniated intervertebral disc
HIDA	hepatobiliary iminodiacetic acid
HIE, HIX	Health Information Exchange
HIM	health information management; Health Insurance Marketplace
HIMSS	Health Information Management System Society
HIPAA	Health Insurance Portability and Accountability Act
HIPDB	Healthcare Integrity and Protection Data Bank
H-ISAC	Health Information Sharing and Analysis Center
HISP	Health Information Service Provider
HIT	health information technology; heparin-induced thrombocytopenia
HITECH Act	Health Information Technology for Economic and Clinical Health Act
HIV	human immunodeficiency virus

HIX, HIE	Health Information Exchange
HJR	hepatojugular reflux
HL	hearing level; hearing loss; hepatic lipase; Hodgkin's lymphoma; hyperlipidemia
HLA	histocompatibility locus antigen; human leukocyte antigen; human lymphocyte antigen
HLD, HL	hyperlipidemia
HLHS	hypoplastic left heart syndrome
HLQAT	Hospital Leadership and Quality Assessment Tool
HM	hand movement
HMD	hyaline membrane disease
HMO	health maintenance organization
HMS	hyperreactive malarial splenomegaly
HMSN	hereditary motor sensory neuropathy
HN	hemagglutinin-neuraminidase
H&N	head and neck
HNC	head and neck cancer
HNP	herniated nucleus pulposus
HNPCC	hereditary nonpolyposis colon cancer
HNV	has not voided
h/o, HO	history of
HOA	hypertrophic osteoarthropathy
HOB	head of bed
HOCM	hypertrophic obstructive cardiomyopathy
HOH	hard of hearing
HONK	hyperosmolar non-ketotic
HOPD	hospital outpatient department
hor, hr	hour (hora)

hor decub, hd	at bedtime (hora decubitus)
hor som, hs*	at bedtime (hora somni)*
hosp	hospital
HP	hot pack
H&P	history and physical
HPA	hypothalamic-pituitary-adrenal (axis); hypothalamic-pituitary axis
HPC	hematopoietic progenitor cell; human progenitor cell
HPF	high-power field
HPI	history of present illness
hPL	human placental lactogen
HPLC	high-performance liquid chromatography
HPN, HTN, HT	hypertension
HPNA	Hospice and Palliative Nurses Association
HPOA	hypertrophic pulmonary osteoarthropathy
HPPD	hours per patient day
HPS	hantavirus pulmonary syndrome; hypertrophic pyloric stenosis
HPSA	Health Professional Shortage Area
HPV	human papillomavirus
HQA	Hospital Quality Alliance
HQI	Hospital Quality Initiative
HR	health realization; heart rate
hr, hor	hour (hora)
HRA	health risk assessment
HRCT	high-resolution computed tomography
HRET	Health Research and Educational Trust; Hospital Research and Educational Trust

HRHS	hypoplastic right heart syndrome
HRIG	human rabies immune globulin
HRP	high-risk pool
HRQOL	health-related quality of life
HRS	hepatorenal syndrome
HRSA	Health Resources and Services Administration
HRSD, HAM-D	Hamilton Rating Scale for Depression
HRT	hormone replacement therapy
HS*	half strength*; herpes simplex
hs*, hor som	at bedtime (hora somni)*
HSA	health savings account; Health Services Administration
HSCT	hematopoietic stem cell transplantation
HSG	herpes simplex genitalis; hysterosalpingogram; hysterosalpingography
HSIL, HGSIL	high-grade squamous intraepithelial lesion
HSM	hepatosplenomegaly
HSP	Henoch-Schönlein purpura
HSRV	hospital-specific relative value
HSV	herpes simplex virus; hypersensitivity vasculitis
HSV-1	herpes simplex virus type 1
HSV-2	herpes simplex virus type 2
HT	Histotechnician; hormone therapy; hypertension
HTL	Histotechnologist
HTLV	human T-lymphotropic virus
HTN, HPN, HT	hypertension
HU	Hounsfield unit
HUB	hyperactive urinary bladder
HUS	hemolytic uremic syndrome

husb	husband
HV	home visit; hypersensitivity vasculitis
HVA	homovanillic acid
HVD	hypertensive vascular disease
Hx	history
hyg	hygiene
hyper	above/high/over
hypo	below/low/under; hypodermic
hyst	hysterectomy
Hz	hertz
HZV	herpes zoster virus
I	iodine
IA	incidental appendectomy; intra-amniotic; intra-aortic; intra-arterial; intra-articular
IAA	insulin autoantibody
IABP	intra-aortic balloon pump
IAC	internal auditory canal
IADL	instrumental activity of daily living
IAI	intra-amniotic infection
IANB	inferior alveolar nerve block
IAW	in accordance with
IBC*	inflammatory breast cancer*; invasive breast cancer*; iron-binding capacity
IBCLC	International Board Certified Lactation Consultant
IBD	inflammatory bowel disease
IBM	inclusion body myositis
IBS	irritable bowel syndrome
IBW	ideal body weight

IC	immunocompromised; infection control; informed consent; immune complex; inspiratory capacity; intensive care; interstitial cystitis; ischemic cardiomyopathy; intracavitary; intracardiac
ICCE	intracapsular cataract extraction
ICCU	intensive coronary care unit
ICD	implantable cardiac defibrillator; implantable cardioverter defibrillator; intercostal chest drain; International Classification of Diseases
ICDS	Integrated Child Development Services
ICER	incremental cost-effectiveness ratio
ICF	intermediate care facility; intracellular fluid
ICG	impedance cardiogram; impedance cardiography
ICH	intracerebral hemorrhage
ICM, ICMP, IC	ischemic cardiomyopathy
ICN	International Council of Nurses
ICP	integrated care partnership; integrated care provider; intracranial pressure
ICPM	intracranial pressure monitoring
ICS	inhaled corticosteroid; intercostal space
ICSH	interstitial cell-stimulating hormone
ICSI	intracytoplasmic sperm injection
ICU	intensive care unit
ID	identification; immunodiffusion; infectious disease; infective dose; intradermal
id	the same (idem)
I&D*	incision and drainage*; irrigation and debridement*

IDA	iron deficiency anemia
IDC	indwelling catheter; invasive ductal carcinoma
IDCM	idiopathic dilated cardiomyopathy
IDD	insulin-dependent diabetes
IDDM	insulin-dependent diabetes mellitus
IDL	intermediate-density lipoprotein
IDM	infant of diabetic mother
IDR	idiosyncratic drug reaction
IDT	interdisciplinary team
IDU	injection drug user
IE	infective endocarditis
I:E ratio	inspiratory to expiratory ratio
IEF	isoelectric focusing
IEM	inborn errors of metabolism
IEN	intraepithelial neoplasia
IF	immunofluorescence; intrinsic factor
IFA	immunofluorescence assay
IFC	interferential current
IFE	immunofixation electrophoresis
IFG	impaired fasting glucose
IFN	interferon
IFRT	involved-field radiation therapy
Ig	immunoglobulin
IgA, IgD, etc.	immunoglobulin A, immunoglobulin D, etc.
IGF	insulin-like growth factor
IGH	idiopathic guttate hypomelanosis; impaired glucose homeostasis
IGIV	immune globulin intravenous
IGRA	interferon gamma release assay

IGT	impaired glucose tolerance
IH	infectious hepatitis; inguinal hernia
IHC	immunohistochemistry
IHD	ischemic heart disease
IHI	Institute for Healthcare Improvement
IHPS	infantile hypertrophic pyloric stenosis
IHSS	idiopathic hypertrophic subaortic stenosis
II	intellectual impairment
IID	intermittent infusion device
IIEF	International Index of Erectile Function
IIF	indirect immunofluorescence
IJ*	injection*; internal jugular
IL	indirect laryngoscopy; interleukin
ILAR	International League of Associations for Rheumatology
ILD	interstitial lung disease
ILI	influenza-like illness
IM	infectious mononucleosis; internal medicine; intramedullary; intramuscular
IMA	inferior mesenteric artery; internal mammary artery
IMB	intermenstrual bleeding
IMC	intermediate care
IMCU	intermediate care unit
IMG	International Medical Graduate
IMI	intramuscular injection
IMM	intramyometrial
imm	immunization
immed	immediate/immediately

imp	impression
IMPACT Act	Improving Medicare Post-Acute Care Transformation Act
impair	impaired/impairment
IMRT	intensity-modulated radiation therapy; intensity-modulated radiotherapy
IMT	immunotherapy; inflammatory myofibroblastic tumor; intima-media thickness
IMV	intermittent mandatory ventilation
IN*	intranasal*
in	inch
in utero	in the uterus
in vitro	in glass; in the laboratory
in vivo	in the living body
inc	incomplete; incontinent
incr	increase
IND	investigational new drug
ind	independent; individual; induction
indic	indicate/indication
inf	infant; infection; inferior; infusion
inflam	inflammation
inh, inhal	inhaled/inhalation
inhib	inhibitor
inj	inject/injection; injury
inpt, IP	inpatient
INR	international normalized ratio
INS	Infusion Nurses Society
ins	insurance
inst	institution; instructed/instruction; instrument

instill	instillation
insuff	insufficient
INT	intermittent needle therapy
int	interior; intermittent; internal
int rot, IR	internal rotation
inv	inversion
invol	involuntary
IO	intraosseous
I&O	intake and output
IOC	intraoperative cholangiogram; intraoperative cholangiography
IOI	intraosseous infusion
IOL	induction of labor; intraocular lens
IOM	Institute of Medicine
IOP	intensive outpatient program; intraocular pressure
IOV	initial office visit
IP	inpatient; interphalangeal; intraperitoneal
IPA	Independent Practice Association; Independent Physician Association
IPAP	inspiratory positive airway pressure
IPD	intermittent peritoneal dialysis; interpupillary distance
IPF	idiopathic pulmonary fibrosis; inpatient psychiatric facility
IPG	impedance phlebogram; impedance phlebography; impedance plethysmogram; impedance plethysmography; implantable pulse generator
IPH	idiopathic pulmonary hemosiderosis; intraparenchymal hemorrhage

IPI	International Prognostic Index
IPJ	interphalangeal joint
IPMN	intraductal papillary mucinous neoplasm
IPn	interstitial pneumonia
IPOC	interdisciplinary plan of care
IPP	intermittent positive pressure
IPPA	inspection, palpation, percussion, auscultation
IPPB	intermittent positive pressure breathing
IPPV	intermittent positive pressure ventilation
IPS	idiopathic pneumonia syndrome
IPV	inactivated poliovirus vaccine; intrapulmonary percussive ventilation
IQ	intelligence quotient
IQR	Inpatient Quality Reporting
IR	immediate release; insulin resistance; internal rotation; interventional radiology; Interventional Radiologist
IRB	Institutional Review Board; intern/resident-to-bed ratio; Investigational Review Board
IRBBB	incomplete right bundle branch block
IRCU	intermediate respiratory care unit
IRDM*	insulin-requiring diabetes mellitus*; insulin-resistant diabetes mellitus*
IRDS	infant respiratory distress syndrome
IRF	inpatient rehabilitation facility
IRIDA	iron-refractory iron deficiency anemia
IRIS	immune reconstitution inflammatory syndrome
irreg	irregular
irrig	irrigate/irrigation

IRS	identical, related, or similar
IRV	inspiratory reserve volume
IS	incentive spirometry; intercostal space
ISA	intrinsic sympathomimetic activity
ISG	immune serum globulin
iSGS, ISS	idiopathic subglottic stenosis
ISH	isolated systolic hypertension
ISMP	Institute for Safe Medication Practices
ISO	International Organization for Standardization
isol	isolation
ISQ	no change (in status quo)
ISR	immune status ratio
IST	inappropriate sinus tachycardia
IT*	immature teratoma; intrathecal*; intratracheal*
ITB	iliotibial band
ITBS	iliotibial band syndrome
ITP	idiopathic thrombocytopenic purpura; immune thrombocytopenic purpura
ITT	insulin tolerance test; intent-to-treat
ITU	intensive therapy unit; intensive treatment unit
IU*	international unit*
IUCD	intrauterine contraceptive device
IUD	intrauterine device
IUFD	intrauterine fetal death; intrauterine fetal demise; intrauterine fetal distress
IUGR	intrauterine growth restriction
IUI	intrauterine insemination
IUO	investigational use only
IUP	intrauterine pregnancy

IUPC	intrauterine pressure catheter
IUS	intrauterine system
IUT	intrauterine transfusion
IV	intravenous; intraventricular
IVAD	intravenous access device
IVC	inferior vena cava; intravenous cholangiogram; intravenous cholangiography
IVCD	intraventricular conduction delay
IVD	in vitro diagnostics; intervertebral disk
IVDA	intravenous drug abuse
IVDD	intervertebral disk disease
IVDU	intravenous drug use
IVE	intravascular embolization
IVF	in vitro fertilization; intravascular fluid; intravenous feeding; intravenous fluid
IVH	intravenous hyperalimentation; intraventricular hemorrhage
IVIg	intravenous immunoglobulin
IVP	intravenous push; intravenous pyelogram; intravenous pyelography
IVPB	intravenous piggyback
IVPG	intravenous pyogenic granuloma
IVRA	intravenous regional anesthesia
IVU	intravenous urogram; intravenous urography
IVUS	intravascular ultrasound
IV&V	independent verification and validation
IWMI	inferior wall myocardial infarction
IXT	intermittent exotropia
J	joule

JCA	juvenile chronic arthritis; juvenile cystic adenomyoma
JCAHO	Joint Commission on Accreditation of Healthcare Organizations
JCV	JC (John Cunningham) virus
JDM	juvenile dermatomyositis; juvenile diabetes mellitus
JEV	Japanese encephalitis virus
JIA	juvenile idiopathic arthritis
JOD	juvenile-onset diabetes
JODM	juvenile-onset diabetes mellitus
JPD, JP	Jackson-Pratt drain
JR	junctional rhythm
JRA	juvenile rheumatoid arthritis
jt, jnt	joint
J-tube	jejunostomy tube
juv	juvenile
JVD	jugular vein distention
JVP	jugular venous pressure; jugular venous pulse
K	potassium
KA	ketoacidosis
KAFO	knee-ankle-foot orthosis
KB	ketone bodies; knee brace
Kcal, Cal, C	Kilocalorie
KCS	keratoconjunctivitis sicca
KCT	kaolin clotting time
KD	Kawasaki disease
KDA	known drug allergy
kDa	kilodalton

kDNA	kinetoplast DNA
KELS	Kohlman Evaluation of Living Skills
kg	kilogram
kHz	kilohertz
KJ	knee jerk
KLS	kidney, liver, spleen
KO	keep open
KOR	keep open rate
kPa	kilopascal
KPC	Klebsiella pneumoniae carbapenemase
KS	Kaposi sarcoma; Kartagener syndrome
KSHV	Kaposi sarcoma-associated herpesvirus
KUB	kidney, ureter, bladder
kV	kilovolt
KVO	keep vein open
L	liter
L1, L2, etc.	lumbar vertebrae (first, second, etc.)
LA	lactic acid; lactic acidosis; laser angioplasty; left arm; left atrial; left atrium; long-acting; lupus anticoagulant; lymphadenopathy; local anesthetic
L&A	light and accommodation
LAA	left atrial appendage
lab	laboratory
LABA	long-acting beta agonist
LAC	live and active culture; long arm cast; lupus anticoagulant
lac	laceration
lact	lactate/lactating

LAD	left anterior descending (artery); left axis deviation; leukocyte adhesion deficiency; lymphadenopathy
LAE	left atrial enlargement
LAFB	left anterior fascicular block
LAH, LAHB	left anterior hemiblock
LAIV	live attenuated influenza vaccine
LAK	lymphokine-activated killer (cell)
LAM	lactation amenorrhea method
LAO	left anterior oblique
LAP	leukocyte alkaline phosphatase; left atrial pressure
lap	laparoscopy; laparotomy
LAR	low anterior resection
LARP	left anterior, right posterior
LAS	lymphadenopathy syndrome
LASER	light amplification by stimulated emission of radiation
LASIK	laser-assisted in situ keratomileusis
lat	lateral
LATS	long-acting thyroid stimulator
LAVH	laparoscopic assisted vaginal hysterectomy
lax	laxative
LB	large bowel; live birth; lower body
lb	pound
L&B	laryngoscopy and bronchoscopy
LBBB	left bundle branch block
LBD	Lewy body dementia
LBO	large bowel obstruction

LBP	low back pain; lower back pain; low blood pressure
LBW	low birth weight
LC	laparoscopic cholecystectomy
LCA	left coronary artery
LCIS	lobular carcinoma in situ
LCL	lateral collateral ligament
LCM	left costal margin; lymphocytic choriomeningitis
LC-MS	liquid chromatography-mass spectrometry
LCMV	lymphocytic choriomeningitis virus
LCPD	Legg-Calve-Perthes disease
LCSW	Licensed Clinical Social Worker
LCV	leukocytoclastic vasculitis
LCX	left circumflex artery
LD	learning disability; left deltoid; lethal dose; Lyme disease
L&D	labor and delivery
LDH	lactate dehydrogenase
LDL	low-density lipoprotein
LDR	labor, delivery, recovery
LDRP	labor, delivery, recovery, postpartum
LE	left eye; leukocyte esterase; lower extremity; lupus erythematosus
LEEP	loop electrosurgical excision procedure
LEP	laparoscopic extraperitoneal; limited English proficiency
LES	lower esophageal sphincter
LET	lidocaine-epinephrine-tetracaine
LFA	left forearm; left frontoanterior

LFD*	lactose-free diet*; low-fat diet*; low-fiber diet*
LFP	left frontoposterior
LFT	left frontotransverse; letter fluency test; liver function test
lg	large
LGA	large for gestational age
LGI	lower gastrointestinal
LGL	Lown-Ganong-Levine
LGSIL, LSIL	low-grade squamous intraepithelial lesion
LGV	lymphogranuloma venereum
LH	left hand; lightheaded; luteinizing hormone
LHC	left heart catheterization
LHF	left heart failure
LHRH	luteinizing hormone-releasing hormone
Li	lithium
LIF	leukemia inhibitory factor
lig	ligament
LIH	left inguinal hernia
LIMA	left internal mammary artery
LIQ	lower inner quadrant
liq	liquid
LITT	laser-induced interstitial thermotherapy; laser interstitial thermal therapy
LKS	liver, kidney, spleen
LL*	left lateral; left leg*; left lung*
LLB	long leg brace
LLC	long leg cast
LLD	leg length discrepancy; limb length discrepancy
LLE	left lower extremity

LLETZ	large loop excision of the transformation zone
LLL	left lower lobe
LLN	lower limits of normal
LLQ	left lower quadrant
LLSB	left lower sternal border
LMA	laryngeal mask airway; left mentoanterior
LMCA	left main coronary artery
LMHC	Licensed Mental Health Counselor
LML	left mediolateral; left middle lobe
LMN	Letter of Medical Necessity; lower motor neuron
LMO	living modified organism
LMP	last menstrual period; low malignant potential
LMS	leiomyosarcoma
LMT	left mentotransverse
LN	liquid nitrogen; lymph node
LND	lymph node dissection
LNI	lymph node involvement
LNMP	last normal menstrual period
LOA	leave of absence; left occiput anterior; level of activity; loss of appetite; lysis of adhesions
LOB	loss of balance
LOC	laxative of choice; level of consciousness; loss of consciousness
LoF	loss of function
LOH	loss of heterozygosity
LOI	loss of imprinting
LOL	lymph obligatory load
LOM	limitation of motion; loss of motion; limitation of movement; loss of movement

LOP	left occiput posterior
LOQ	lower outer quadrant
LOR	loss of resistance
LOS	length of stay
LOT	left occiput transverse
LP	lumbar puncture
LPD	luteal phase defect; luteal phase deficiency
LPFB	left posterior fascicular block
LPI	laser peripheral iridotomy
LPL	lipoprotein lipase
LPM	liters per minute
LPN	Licensed Practical Nurse
LPO	left posterior oblique
LPP	lichen planopilaris
LPT	Licensed Physical Therapist
LQ	lower quadrant
LQTS	long QT syndrome
LR	labor room
L&R	left and right
L/R, L-R	left to right
LRI	lower respiratory infection
LRINEC	Laboratory Risk Indicator for Necrotizing Fasciitis
LRS	lower respiratory symptoms
LRT	lower respiratory tract
LRTI	lower respiratory tract infection
LS	lichen sclerosus; lumbosacral; Lynch syndrome
L/S ratio	lecithin to sphingomyelin ratio
LSA	left sacrum anterior; lichen sclerosus et atrophicus

LSB	left sternal border
LSC	left subclavian
LSCS	lower segment cesarean section
LSD	lysergic acid diethylamide
LSIL, LGSIL	low-grade squamous intraepithelial lesion
LSK	liver, spleen, kidney
LSO	left salpingo-oophorectomy
LSP	left sacrum posterior
L-spine	lumbar spine
LST	laterally spreading tumor; left sacrum transverse
LT	leukotriene; light touch
lt	left
LTAC	long-term acute care
LTB	laryngotracheobronchitis
LTC	long-term care; long-term condition
LTCF	long-term care facility
LTCH	long-term care hospital
LTCS	low transverse cesarean section
LTD	long-term disability
LTE	less than effective; life-threatening event
LTL	laparoscopic tubal ligation
LTM	long-term memory
LTR	laryngotracheal reconstruction
LTV	long-term variability
ltx	latex
L&U	lower and upper
LUA	left upper arm
LUD	left uterine displacement
LUE	left upper extremity

LUL	left upper lobe
LUQ	left upper quadrant
LUS	lower uterine segment
LUTS	lower urinary tract symptoms
LV	left ventricle; live vaccine
LVA	left ventricular aneurysm
LVAD	left ventricular assist device
LVE	left ventricular enlargement
LVEDP	left ventricular end-diastolic pressure
LVEF	left ventricular ejection fraction
LVET	left ventricular ejection time
LVF	left ventricular failure; left ventricular function
LVG	left ventriculogram; left ventriculography
LVH	left ventricular hypertrophy
lvl	level
LVN	Licensed Vocational Nurse
LVOT	left ventricular outflow tract
LVOTO	left ventricular outflow tract obstruction
LVP	large volume paracentesis
LVPW	left ventricular posterior wall
LVSD	left ventricular systolic dysfunction
LVSV	left ventricular stroke volume
L&W	living and well
LWBS	left without being seen
LWD	living with disease
LWDII	lost workday injury and illness
LWOT	left without treatment
LX	larynx
LXT	left exotropia

lym, lymphs	lymphocytes
lytes	electrolytes
m	meter
MA	medical assistance; Medicare Advantage; mental age
mA	milliampere
mAb, moAb	monoclonal antibody
MABP	mean arterial blood pressure
MAC	Medicare Administrative Contractor; monitored anesthesia care; Mycobacterium avium complex
MACE	major adverse cardiac event; major adverse cardiovascular event
MACRA	Medicare Access and CHIP Reauthorization Act
MAE	moves all extremities
MAFO	molded ankle-foot orthosis
mag, Mg	magnesium
MAHA	microangiopathic hemolytic anemia
MAI	Mycobacterium avium-intracellulare
MAL	midaxillary line
MALT	mucosa-associated lymphoid tissue
MAMC	midarm muscle circumference
man prim	first thing in the morning (mane primum)
mand	mandatory; mandible/mandibular
mane	in the morning
MANOS	minilaparoscopy-assisted natural orifice surgery
MAO	monoamine oxidase
MAOI	monoamine oxidase inhibitor
MAP	mean airway pressure; mean arterial pressure
MAR	Medication Administration Record

MAS	meconium aspiration syndrome; mobile arm support
MAST	Michigan Alcohol Screening Test; medical anti-shock trousers; military anti-shock trousers
mast, Mx	mastectomy
MAT	medication-assisted treatment; microscopic agglutination test; Miller Analogies Test; modular antigen transporter; multifocal atrial tachycardia
max	maxilla; maxillary; maximum
MBBS	Bachelor of Medicine, Bachelor of Surgery
MBC	maximum breathing capacity; metastatic breast cancer
MBD	minimal brain dysfunction
MBSS	modified barium swallow study
MBU	mother and baby unit
MC	metacarpal
mc, mCi	millicurie
MCA	middle cerebral artery; motorcycle accident; mucinous cystadenoma
MCAD	medium-chain acyl-CoA dehydrogenase
MCAT	Medical College Admission Test
MCC	major complication or comorbidity; motorcycle collision
MCD	minimal change disease; multiple carboxylase deficiency
MCF	macrophage chemotactic factor; middle cranial fossa
mcg	microgram
mcgtt	microdrop

MCH	mean cell hemoglobin; mean corpuscular hemoglobin
MCHB	Maternal and Child Health Bureau
MCHC	mean corpuscular hemoglobin concentration
MCI	mild cognitive impairment
mCi, mc	millicurie
MCL	medial collateral ligament; midclavicular line
mcL, µL	microliter
MCM	medical countermeasure
MCO	managed care organization
MCP	managed care plan; metacarpophalangeal
MCPJ, MPJ	metacarpophalangeal joint
MC&S	microscopy, culture, and sensitivity
MCTD	mixed connective tissue disease
MCV	mean cell volume; mean corpuscular volume
MD	Doctor of Medicine; medical doctor; Meniere's disease; muscular dystrophy
MDA	medical device alert
MDC	Major Diagnostic Category
MDCT	multidetector computed tomography
MDD	major depressive disorder; maximum daily dose
MDE	major depressive episode
MDH	Medicare-dependent hospital
MDI	metered-dose inhaler
MDISS	Medical Device Innovation, Safety, and Security Consortium
mdnt, mn	midnight
MDR	multidrug resistant; multiple drug resistance
MDR-TB	multidrug-resistant tuberculosis

MDS	Minimum Data Set; myelodysplastic syndrome
MDT	multidisciplinary team
MD-VIPER	Medical Device Vulnerability Intelligence Program for Evaluation and Response
ME	Medical Examiner; muscle energy; myalgic encephalomyelitis
M/E ratio	myeloid to erythroid ratio
MEA	multiple endocrine adenomatosis
MEC	moderately emetogenic chemotherapy
MED	minimal erythema dose; minimum effective dose
med	medial; medical; medication; medicine
Medigap	Medicare Supplement Insurance
MEDLINE	Medical Literature Analysis and Retrieval System Online
MedPAC	Medicare Payment Advisory Commission
MedPAR	Medicare Provider Analysis and Review
MEE	middle ear effusion
MEFR	maximum expiratory flow rate
MEG	magnetoencephalogram; magnetoencephalography
MELD	Model for End-Stage Liver Disease
mem	member; memory
MEN	multiple endocrine neoplasia
MEPS	Medical Expenditure Panel Survey
mEq	milliequivalent
MeSH	Medical Subject Headings
MET	Medical Emergency Team; metabolic equivalent of task
metab	metabolic; metabolism

mets	metastasis
M&F	mother and father
MFC	medial femoral condyle
MFFD	medically fit for discharge
MFM	maternal-fetal medicine
MG	myasthenia gravis
Mg, mag	magnesium
mg	milligram
MGF	maternal grandfather
MGM	maternal grandmother
MGN	membranous glomerulonephritis
MGUS	monoclonal gammopathy of undetermined significance
MH	malignant hyperthermia; medical history; mental health
MHC	major histocompatibility complex; mental health center
MHE	mental health evaluation
MHPAEA	Mental Health Parity and Addiction Equity Act
MHR	maternal heart rate; maximum heart rate
MHT	Mental Health Therapist
MHU	mental health unit
MHx, MH	medical history
MHz	megahertz
MI	mental illness; mitral insufficiency; myocardial infarction
MIBI	sestamibi
MIC	minimum inhibitory concentration
MICA	mentally ill chemical abuser

MI/CD	mentally ill/chemically dependent
MICU	medical intensive care unit; mobile intensive care unit
MID	mentally ill and dangerous; minimum infective dose; multi-infarct dementia
mid	middle
MIDCAB	minimally invasive direct coronary artery bypass
MIF	melanocyte-inhibiting factor; Müllerian inhibitory factor
min	minimum; minute
MIP	maximum intensity projection
MIPPA	Medicare Improvements for Patients and Providers Act
MIPS	Merit-Based Incentive Payment System
MIS	minimally invasive surgery; Müllerian inhibiting substance
misc	miscellaneous
mist	mixture (mistura)
MIT	Medical Imaging Technician
mJ	millijoule
ML	midline
mL	milliliter
MLBW	moderately low birth weight
MLC	midline catheter; multilumen catheter
MLD	minimum lethal dose
MLE	mediolateral episiotomy
MLF	medial longitudinal fasciculus
MLPA	multiplex ligation-dependent probe amplification
MLR	medical loss ratio; mixed lymphocyte reaction

MLT	macular laser therapy; Medical Laboratory Technician
MM	malignant melanoma; million; mucous membrane; multiple myeloma; muscle mass; myeloid metaplasia
mm	millimeter
M&M	morbidity and mortality
MMA	Medicare Prescription Drug, Improvement, and Modernization Act; methylmalonic acid; middle meningeal artery
MMEF	maximal mid-expiratory flow
MMEFR	maximal mid-expiratory flow rate
MMF	maxillomandibular fixation
MMI	maximum medical improvement
MMK	Marshall-Marchetti-Krantz (procedure)
MMM	myelofibrosis with myeloid metaplasia
MMMT	malignant mixed Müllerian tumor
mmol	millimole
MMP	Medical Monitoring Project; multiple medical problems
MMPI	Minnesota Multiphasic Personality Inventory
MMR	measles, mumps, rubella (vaccine); mismatch repair
MMRV	measles, mumps, rubella, varicella (vaccine)
MMSE	Mini-Mental State Examination
MMT	malignant mesenchymal tumor; manual muscle test; methadone maintenance treatment
MMWR	Morbidity and Mortality Weekly Report
MN	membranous nephropathy
mn, mdnt	midnight

MND	motor neuron disease
MNT	medical nutrition therapy
mo	month
moAb, mAb	monoclonal antibody
MOB	mother of baby
mod	moderate; modified
MODY	maturity-onset diabetes of the young
mol	mole
mol wt, MW	molecular weight
MOLST	Medical Orders for Life-Sustaining Treatment
MoM	Milk of Magnesia; multiples of the median
mono	monocyte; mononucleosis
mor dict	as directed (more dicto)
mor sol	in the usual manner (more solito)
mOsm	milliosmole
MP	menstrual pain; menstrual period; midplane; metacarpophalangeal
mPAP	mean pulmonary artery pressure
MPC	maximum permitted concentration; mucopurulent cervicitis
MPD	main pancreatic duct; multiple personality disorder; myeloproliferative disorder
MPFS	Medicare Physician Fee Schedule
MPGN	membranoproliferative glomerulonephritis
MPH	Master of Public Health
MPJ, MCPJ	metacarpophalangeal joint
MPN	most probable number
MPO	myeloperoxidase
MPT	multiprofessional team

MPV	mean platelet volume
MQSA	Mammography Quality Standards Act
MR	medical record; menstrual regulation; mental retardation; mitral regurgitation; modified release
MRA	magnetic resonance angiogram; magnetic resonance angiography
MRCP	magnetic resonance cholangiopancreatogram; magnetic resonance cholangiopancreatography
MRD	medical records department; multiple rising dose
MRgFUS	magnetic resonance guided focused ultrasound
MRI	magnetic resonance imaging
mRNA	messenger RNA
MRS	magnetic resonance spectroscopy
mRS	Modified Rankin Scale
MRSA	methicillin-resistant Staphylococcus aureus
MRSE	methicillin-resistant Staphylococcus epidermidis
MS*	mass spectrometry; mass spectroscopy; mental status; mitral stenosis*; multiple sclerosis*; muscle strength; musculoskeletal
MSA	medical savings account
MSAFP	maternal serum alpha-fetoprotein
MSDS	Material Safety Data Sheet
MSDU	medical surgical day unit
MSE	mental status examination
MSG	monosodium glutamate
MSH	melanocyte-stimulating hormone
MSI	magnetic source imaging
MSK	medullary sponge kidney; musculoskeletal

MSL	midsternal line
MSN	Master of Science in Nursing
MSOF	multisystem organ failure
MSP	Medicare Secondary Payer
MSSA	methicillin-sensitive Staphylococcus aureus
MST	multisystemic therapy
MSU	midstream specimen of urine; monosodium urate
MSUD	maple syrup urine disease
MSW	Master of Social Work; Medical Social Worker
MT	Medical Technologist
Mtb	Mycobacterium tuberculosis
MT-BC	Music Therapist-Board Certified
MTBI	mild traumatic brain injury
MTC	medullary thyroid cancer
MTD	maximum tolerated dose; month-to-date
MTP	metatarsophalangeal
mU	milliunit
mµ	millimicron
MUA	Medically Underserved Area
MUA/P	Medically Underserved Area/Population
MUCP	maximum urethral closure pressure
MUD	matched unrelated donor
MUFA	monounsaturated fatty acid
MUGA	multigated acquisition (scan)
mult	multiple
MUP	Medically Underserved Population
MUS	medically unexplained symptoms
musc	muscle/muscular

MV*	mechanical ventilation*; mitral valve*
mV	millivolt
MVA	motor vehicle accident
MVC	motor vehicle collision; motor vehicle crash
MVI	multivitamin injection
MVIC	maximum voluntary isometric contraction
MVP	mitral valve prolapse
MVR	mitral valve regurgitation; mitral valve repair; mitral valve replacement
MVS	mitral valve stenosis
MVV	maximum ventilatory volume; maximum voluntary ventilation
MW, mol wt	molecular weight
Mx, mast	mastectomy
NA	Nurse Aide; Nursing Assistant
Na	sodium
n/a	not applicable; not available
NAAT	nucleic acid amplification test
NABCO	National Alliance of Breast Cancer Organizations
NABS*	no active bowel sounds*; normal active bowel sounds*
NACHRI	National Association of Children's Hospitals and Related Institutions
NAD	no acute disease; no apparent distress; no appreciable disease; nothing abnormal detected
NAF	notice of adverse findings
NAFLD	non-alcoholic fatty liver disease
NAHC	National Association for Home Care and Hospice
NAI	no action indicated

NAM	National Academy of Medicine
NAMCS	National Ambulatory Medical Care Survey
NAS	intranasal; neonatal abstinence syndrome; no added salt
NASG	non-pneumatic anti-shock garment
NASH	non-alcoholic steatohepatitis
NAT	non-accidental trauma; nucleic acid test
NB	newborn
nb	note well (nota bene)
NBHS	newborn hearing screen
NBIA	neurodegeneration with brain iron accumulation
NBN	newborn nursery
NBT	nitroblue tetrazolium
NBTE	nonbacterial thrombotic endocarditis
NBTNF/M	newborn, term, normal, female/male
n/c, NC	no complaints
NC/AT	normocephalic/atraumatic
NCCM, NCC	noncompaction cardiomyopathy
NCCN	National Comprehensive Cancer Network
NCCS	National Coalition for Cancer Survivorship
NCEP	National Cholesterol Education Program
NCHS	National Center for Health Statistics
NCI	National Cancer Institute
nCi	nanocurie
NCP	nursing care plan
NCPAP	nasal continuous positive airway pressure
NCQA	National Committee for Quality Assurance
NCS	nerve conduction study
NCV	nerve conduction velocity

NCVHS	National Committee on Vital and Health Statistics
ND	neck dissection; nondistended; normal delivery; not diagnosed
NDA	New Drug Application; non-disclosure agreement
NDC	National Drug Code
NDI	Neck Disability Index; nephrogenic diabetes insipidus
nDNA	native DNA
NE*	neurological examination; norepinephrine; not evaluated*; not examined*
NEAD	non-epileptic attack disorder
NEAP	net endogenous acid production
neb	nebulizer
NEC	necrotizing enterocolitis; not elsewhere classifiable; not elsewhere classified
NED	no evidence of disease
neg	negative
NEL	non-elective
neo	neoplasm
NES	not elsewhere specified
neuro	neurology; Neurologist
NF	National Formulary; neurofibromatosis
NFA	Nursing Facility Administrator
NFLP	non-fasting lipid panel
NFP	natural family planning
NFR	not for resuscitation
NG	nasogastric
ng	nanogram

NGF	nerve growth factor
NGS	next-generation sequencing; neurogenetic syndrome
NGT	nasogastric tube; normal glucose tolerance
NGTD	negative to date; no growth to date
NGU	non-gonococcal urethritis
NH	nursing home
NHAMCS	National Hospital Ambulatory Medical Care Survey
NHANES	National Health and Nutrition Examination Survey
NHC	National Health Council
NHDR	National Healthcare Disparities Report
NHeLP	National Health Law Program
NHIC	National Health Information Center
NHIS	National Health Interview Survey
NHL	non-Hodgkin's lymphoma
NHOPI	Native Hawaiian or Other Pacific Islander
NHP	nursing home placement
NHPC	National Health Plan Collaborative
NHQI	Nursing Home Quality Initiative
NHQR	National Healthcare Quality Report
NHS	normal human serum
NHSN	National Healthcare Safety Network
NHW	non-healing wound
NI	not indicated
NIBP	non-invasive blood pressure
NIC	neonatal intensive care
NICM, NICMP	nonischemic cardiomyopathy

NICU	neonatal intensive care unit
NIDDM	non-insulin-dependent diabetes mellitus
NIF	negative inspiratory force
NIH	National Institutes of Health
NIHSS	National Institutes of Health Stroke Scale
NILM	negative for intraepithelial lesion or malignancy
NINR	National Institute of Nursing Research
NIOSH	National Institute for Occupational Safety and Health
NIPPV	nasal intermittent positive pressure ventilation; non-invasive positive pressure ventilation
NIS	National Immunization Survey
NK	natural killer (cell); not known
NKA	no known allergies
NKDA	no known drug allergies
NKFA	no known food allergies
NKH, NKHG	nonketotic hyperglycinemia
nL	nanoliter
nl, norm	normal
NLAAS	National Latino and Asian American Study
NLN	National League for Nursing
NLP	no light perception
NLT	not less than
NM	neuromuscular; not monitored; nuclear medicine
nm	nanometer
NMDA	N-methyl D-aspartate
NMJ	neuromuscular junction
nmol	nanomole

NMR	nuclear magnetic resonance
NMS	neuroleptic malignant syndrome
NMT	not more than
NNH	number needed to harm
NNP	Neonatal Nurse Practitioner
NNRTI	non-nucleoside reverse transcriptase inhibitor
NNT	number needed to treat
NNU	neonatal unit
no, num	number
noct	at night (nocte)
noct maneq	at night and in the morning (nocte maneque)
NOE	nasoorbitoethmoid
NOF	neck of femur
NOMI	non-occlusive mesenteric ischemia
NORD	National Organization for Rare Disorders
NOS	nitric oxide synthase; not otherwise specified
NP	nasopharyngeal; neuropsychiatric; neuropsychology; Neuropsychologist; Nurse Practitioner
NPA	nasal pharyngeal aspirate
NPC	nasopharyngeal carcinoma; non-protein calorie
NPCPAP	nasopharyngeal continuous positive airway pressure
NPDB	National Practitioner Data Bank
NPDR	non-proliferative diabetic retinopathy
NPH	neutral protamine Hagedorn; normal pressure hydrocephalus
NPN	non-protein nitrogen
npo	nothing by mouth (nil per os)
NPPE	negative pressure pulmonary edema

NPPV	noninvasive positive pressure ventilation
NPT	neuropsychological testing; nocturnal penile tumescence
NPV	negative predictive value
NPWT	negative pressure wound therapy
NQF	National Quality Forum
NQWMI	non-Q wave myocardial infarction
NR	no record; no refills; non-reactive
nr, non rep	do not repeat (non repetatur)
NRB	non-rebreather
NRBC	nucleated red blood cell
NRC	normal retinal correspondence
NREM	non-rapid eye movement
NRM	no regular medications; non-rebreathing mask
NRT	nicotine replacement therapy
NRTI	nucleoside reverse transcriptase inhibitor
NS	nervous system; neurological surgery; normal saline; not significant
NSA	National Stroke Association; no significant abnormality
NSAID	nonsteroidal anti-inflammatory drug
NSBB	nonselective beta blocker
NSC	National Safety Council; neural stem cell
NSCLC	non-small cell lung cancer
NSD	normal spontaneous delivery
NSDUH	National Survey on Drug Use and Health
NSE	neuron specific enolase
NSI	nasal saline irrigation
NSICU	neuroscience intensive care unit

NSIP	nonspecific interstitial pneumonia
NSR	nonsignificant risk; normal sinus rhythm
NSS	normal saline solution
NSSP	normal size, shape, position
NST	non-stress test
NSTEMI	non-ST elevation myocardial infarction
NSU	non-specific urethritis
NSV	non-specific vaginitis
NSVD	normal spontaneous vaginal delivery
nsy	nursery
NT	nasotracheal; non-tender; not tested; nuchal translucency
N&T	numbness and tingling
NTD	neural tube defect
NTE	not to exceed
NTM	non-tuberculosis mycobacteria
NTND	non-tender, non-distended
NTS	nucleus tractus solitarius
NTT	nasotracheal tube
NUG	necrotizing ulcerative gingivitis
nullip	nullipara
NUP	necrotizing ulcerative periodontitis
nutr	nutrition
NV	near vision
N&V	nausea and vomiting
NVA	neurovascular assessment
NVD	nausea, vomiting, diarrhea; normal vaginal delivery
NVDC	nausea, vomiting, diarrhea, constipation

NVS	neurological vital sign
NVSS	National Vital Statistics System
N&W	normal and well
NWB	non-weight bearing
NYD	not yet diagnosed
O_2	oxygen
O_2 sat, SaO_2	oxygen saturation
OA	occipital-atlas; occiput anterior; osteoarthritis; osteoarthrosis
OAB	overactive bladder
OAE	otoacoustic emission
OAF	osteoclast activating factor
OAG	open-angle glaucoma
OAT	Office for the Advancement of Telehealth
OAWO	opening abductory wedge osteotomy
OB	obstetrics; Obstetrician
OB/GYN	obstetrics/gynecology; Obstetrician/Gynecologist
obl	oblique
OBS	organic brain syndrome
obs	observe/observation
obst	obstruction
OBUS	obstetric ultrasound
OC	oral contraceptive; osteocalcin
occ	occasional
OCD	obsessive-compulsive disorder
OCE	Outpatient Code Editor
OCG	oral cholecystogram; oral cholecystography
OCP	oral contraceptive pill

OCR	ossicular chain reconstruction
OCT	optical coherence tomography; oxytocin challenge test
OD*	Doctor of Optometry; optical density; overdose; right eye (oculus dexter)*
od	every day (omni die)
ODC	ornithine decarboxylase
ODT	orally disintegrating tablet
OE	otitis externa
O&E	observation and examination
o/e	on examination
OEP	open enrollment period
OFC	occipital-frontal circumference
OG	orogastric
OGT	oral glucose tolerance; orogastric tube
OGTT	oral glucose tolerance test
OH	occupational history; orthostatic hypotension
oh, omn hor	every hour (omni hora)
OHD	organic heart disease
OHL	oral hairy leukoplakia
OHS	obesity hypoventilation syndrome
OHT	orthotopic heart transplantation
OI	opportunistic infection
oint	ointment
ol	oil (oleum)
OLT	orthotopic liver transplant
OM	osteomalacia; osteomyelitis; otitis media
om, omn man	every morning (omni mane)
OMD	organic mental disorder

OME	otitis media with effusion
OMH	Office of Minority Health
OMP	outer membrane protein
OMS	opsoclonus-myoclonus syndrome
ON	optic neuritis; overnight
on	every night (omni nocte)
onc	oncology; Oncologist
ONS	Oncology Nursing Society
OOB	out of bed
OON	out of network
OOP	out of pocket
OP	occiput posterior; opening pressure; outpatient; oropharyngeal; osteoporosis
op	operation; operative
O&P	ova and parasites
OPA	outpatient anesthesia
OPC	outpatient clinic
OPD	outpatient department
OPG	ocular pneumoplethysmogram; ocular pneumoplethysmography
OPH	Office of Public Health
OPHEP	Office of Public Health Emergency Preparedness
OPHS	Office of Public Health and Science
OPMS	oropharyngeal motility study
OPO	Organ Procurement Organization
opp	opposite
OPPT	outpatient physical therapy
OPS	outpatient service; outpatient surgery
OPT	outpatient therapy

opt	optical; optimal
opth	ophthalmology; Ophthalmologist
OPV	oral polio vaccine; outpatient visit
OQR	Outpatient Quality Reporting
OR	odds ratio; operating room
ORHP	Office of Rural Health Policy
ORIF	open reduction and internal fixation
ORL	otorhinolaryngology; Otorhinolaryngologist
ORR	objective response rate
ORS	oral rehydration solution
ORT	oral rehydration therapy
ortho	orthodontic; Orthodontist; orthopedic; Orthopedist; orthostatic
ORTT	Organ Transplant Tracking Record
OS*	left eye (oculus sinister)*; orthopedic surgery; overall survival
OSA	obstructive sleep apnea
OSHA	Occupational Safety and Health Administration
Osm	osmole
OSR	open septorhinoplasty
osteo, os	bone (osteon)
OT	occupational therapy; Occupational Therapist; old tuberculin
OTC	over-the-counter
oto	ear; otolaryngology; Otolaryngologist; otology; Otologist
OTP	opioid treatment program
OTR	Occupational Therapist, Registered
OU*	both eyes (oculi uterque)*

OV	office visit
o/w	otherwise
oz	ounce
$\bar{p}$	after (post)
P2	pulmonic second sound
PA	panic attack; pernicious anemia; physical activity; Physician Assistant; placenta abruption; posterior-anterior; posteroanterior; primary aldosteronism; prior authorization; propionic acidemia; psoriatic arthritis; pulmonary artery
Pa	pascal
P&A	percussion and auscultation
PA view	posteroanterior view
PABA	para-aminobenzoic acid
PAC	premature atrial contraction; pulmonary artery catheter
PA-C	Physician Assistant-Certified
PACE	Program of All-Inclusive Care for the Elderly
$PaCO_2$	partial pressure of arterial carbon dioxide
PACU	post-anesthesia care unit
PAD	peripheral artery disease
PADP	pulmonary artery diastolic pressure
PAF	paroxysmal atrial fibrillation; platelet-activating factor
PAH	phenylalanine hydroxylase; pulmonary arterial hypertension
PAL	peripheral arterial line; posterior axillary line
palp	palpate/palpable/palpation
PALS	Pediatric Advanced Life Support
PAN	polyarteritis nodosa

p-ANCA	perinuclear antineutrophil cytoplasmic antibody
PanCAN	Pancreatic Cancer Action Network
PAO	peak acid output
PaO$_2$	partial pressure of arterial oxygen
PAOD	peripheral artery occlusive disease
PAOP	pulmonary artery occlusion pressure
PAP	patient assistance program; peak airway pressure; positive airway pressure; prescription assistance program; pulmonary alveolar proteinosis; pulmonary arterial pressure
Pap smear	Papanicolaou smear
PAPP-A	pregnancy-associated plasma protein A
PAR	patient at risk; post-anesthesia recovery
para 1, 2, etc.	number of viable births (one, two, etc.)
part vic	divided doses (partes vicibus)
PAS	periodic acid-Schiff
PASARR	Pre-Admission Screening and Annual Resident Review
PASG	pneumatic anti-shock garment
PASH	pseudoangiomatous stromal hyperplasia
PASP	pulmonary artery systolic pressure
PAT	paroxysmal atrial tachycardia; pre-admission testing
path	pathology; Pathologist
PAW	pulmonary artery wedge
PAWP	pulmonary artery wedge pressure
PB	peripheral blood
PBC	primary biliary cholangitis; primary biliary cirrhosis
PBF	partially breastfed; peripheral blood film

PBI	protein-bound iodine
PBM	Pharmacy Benefit Manager
PBPC	peripheral blood progenitor cell
PBSC	peripheral blood stem cell
PBSCT	peripheral blood stem cell transplantation
PBX	probiotic
PC	packed cell; personal care; pressure control
pc	after meals (post cibos)
PCA	patient-controlled analgesia; Patient Care Assistant; Personal Care Assistant
PCa	prostate cancer
PCAP	Prenatal Care Assistance Program
PCC	Poison Control Center; prothrombin complex concentrate
PCCU	pediatric critical care unit
PCD	pneumatic compression device; post-concussion disorder; primary ciliary dyskinesia; primary conduction disease
PCH	personal care home
PChE	pseudocholinesterase
PCI	percutaneous coronary intervention
PCIOL	posterior chamber intraocular lens
PCIP	Pre-Existing Condition Insurance Plan
PCKD, PKD	polycystic kidney disease
PCL	posterior cruciate ligament
PCM	permanent cardiac pacemaker; protein-calorie malnutrition
PCN	penicillin; primary care network
PCNL	percutaneous nephrolithotomy

PCNSL	primary central nervous system lymphoma
PCO	patient complains of; polycystic ovary; primary care office
PCO_2	partial pressure of carbon dioxide
PCOD	polycystic ovary disease
PCORI	Patient-Centered Outcomes Research Institute
PCOS	polycystic ovary syndrome
PCP	phenylcyclohexyl piperidine; Pneumocystis carinii pneumonia; Primary Care Physician; primary care provider
PCR	patient care report; polymerase chain reaction
PCRA	patient-controlled regional analgesia
PCS	pelvic congestion syndrome; post-concussion syndrome
PCT	Patient Care Technician; proximal convoluted tubule; photochemical treatment; progesterone challenge test
pct	percent
PCU*	palliative care unit*; progressive care unit*
PCV	packed cell volume; pneumococcal vaccine; polycythemia vera; pressure control ventilation
PCW	pulmonary capillary wedge
PCWP	pulmonary capillary wedge pressure
PCXR	portable chest x-ray
PD*	panic disorder*; personality disorder*; Parkinson's disease*; Peyronie's disease*; progressive disease; pulmonary disease; prism diopter; peritoneal dialysis; postural drainage; provisional discharge; psychotic depression; pupillary distance

PDA	patent ductus arteriosus; posterior descending artery
PDD	pervasive development disorder
PDE	permitted daily exposure; phosphodiesterase
PDF	portable document format
PDGF	platelet-derived growth factor
PDMP	Prescription Drug Monitoring Program
PDN	Private Duty Nurse
PDP	prescription drug plan
PD&P	postural drainage and percussion
PDPM	Patient Driven Payment Model
PDR	Physicians' Desk Reference; proliferative diabetic retinopathy
pdr, pwdr	powder
PDT	photodynamic therapy
PE	physical examination; pleural effusion; preeclampsia; pulmonary edema; pulmonary embolism
PEA	pulseless electrical activity
PEARL	pupils equal and reactive to light
PED	performance-enhancing drug
ped	pediatric; Pediatrician
PEEP	positive end-expiratory pressure
PEF	peak expiratory flow
PEFR	peak expiratory flow rate
PEG	percutaneous endoscopic gastrostomy; polyethylene glycol; pneumoencephalogram; pneumoencephalography
PEJ	percutaneous endoscopic jejunostomy
PEL	permissible exposure limit

PEM	protein-energy malnutrition
PEMF	pulsing electromagnetic field
PEP	pancreatic enzyme product; positive expiratory pressure; post-exposure prophylaxis
per	for each; period; periodic; through/by
perf	perforation
PERM	progressive encephalomyelitis with rigidity and myoclonus
perm	permanent
peron	peroneal
PERRL	pupils equal, round, reactive to light
PERRLA	pupils equal, round, reactive to light and accommodation
PERS	Personal Emergency Response System
PET	positron emission tomography
PEU	protein-energy undernutrition
PEX, PE, PX	physical examination
PF	plantar flexion
PFC	persistent fetal circulation; plaque-forming cell; prefrontal cortex
PFO	patent foramen ovale
PFP, P4P	pay for performance
PFT	pulmonary function test
PG	phosphatidylglycerol
pg	picogram
PGF	paternal grandfather
PGL	persistent generalized lymphadenopathy; plasma glucose level
PGM	paternal grandmother

PH	parathyroid hormone; past history; pinhole; poor health; pulmonary hypertension; public health
pH	potential of hydrogen; power of hydrogen
PHA	Public Health Advisory
PHAB	Public Health Advisory Board
pharm	pharmacy
PharmD	Doctor of Pharmacy
PHCP	primary healthcare provider
PhD	Doctor of Philosophy
PHG	portal hypertensive gastropathy
PHI	protected health information
PHIN	Public Health Information Network
PHN	postherpetic neuralgia; Public Health Nurse
PHNI	pinhole no improvement
PHO	physician-hospital organization; Public Health Officer
phos	phosphate
PHP	partial hospitalization program
PHQ	Patient Health Questionnaire
PHR	peak heart rate; personal health record
PHS	Public Health Service
PHT	Public Health Technician
PHx, PH	past history
phys	physical; physiology; Physiologist
physio	physiotherapy; Physiotherapist
PI	perfusion index; peripheral iridotomy; present illness; previous illness; protease inhibitor; pulmonic insufficiency

PICC	peripherally inserted central catheter
PICU	pediatric intensive care unit; psychiatric intensive care unit; pulmonary intensive care unit
PID	pelvic inflammatory disease
PIE	plan, intervention, evaluation
PIF	peak inspiratory flow
PIFR	peak inspiratory flow rate
PIH	pregnancy-induced hypertension; prolactin-inhibiting hormone
PII	patient identifiable information; personally identifiable information
PIL	patient information leaflet; PEGylated immunoliposome
pil	pill
PIP	peak inspiratory pressure; periodic interim payment; proximal interphalangeal
PIVC	peripheral intravenous catheter
PJC	premature junctional complex; premature junctional contraction
PJS	Peutz-Jeghers syndrome
PK	protein kinase
P-K test	Prausnitz-Küstner test
PKD, PCKD	polycystic kidney disease
PKP	penetrating keratoplasty
PKR	partial knee replacement
PKU	phenylketonuria
PL	palmaris longus; partial laryngectomy
PLIF	posterior lumbar interbody fusion
PLL	posterior lateral line

PLT, plat	platelet
PM, pm	evening; after noon (post meridiem)
PMB	postmenopausal bleeding
PMD	Primary Medical Doctor; Private Medical Doctor
PMDD	premenstrual dysphoric disorder
PMFSH	past medical, family, social history
PMH, PMHx	past medical history
PMI	point of maximal impulse; private medical insurance
PML	progressive multifocal leukoencephalopathy
PMN	polymorphonuclear neutrophil
PMNL	polymorphonuclear neutrophil leukocyte
pmol	picomole
PMP	previous menstrual period; pseudomyxoma peritonei
PMR	percutaneous myocardial revascularization; proportionate mortality ratio; polymyalgia rheumatica
PM&R	physical medicine and rehabilitation
PMS	premenstrual syndrome
PMT	premenstrual tension
PMU	pain management unit
PN	parenteral nutrition; poorly nourished; Practical Nurse; prenatal; product name; progress note
PNA	partial nail avulsion; percutaneous needle aspiration; pneumonia; postnatal age
PNB, PNBx	prostate needle biopsy
PNC	penicillin; premature nodal contraction; prenatal care
PND	paroxysmal nocturnal dyspnea; postnasal drip

PNET	primitive neuroectodermal tumor
pneu, PNA	pneumonia
PNF	proprioceptive neuromuscular facilitation
PNH	paroxysmal nocturnal hemoglobinuria
PNI	peripheral nerve injury
PNM	perinatal mortality
PNP	Pediatric Nurse Practitioner
PNS	parasympathetic nervous system; peripheral nervous system
PNV	prenatal vitamin
PNX, PTX	pneumothorax
PO	phone order; purchase order
po	by mouth (per os)
PO_2	partial pressure of oxygen
POA	power of attorney; present on admission
POAG	primary open-angle glaucoma
POC	plan of care; point of care; point of contact; products of conception
POD	point of distribution; postoperative day; postoperative delirium
POE	point of entry
POLST	Physician Orders for Life-Sustaining Treatment
PONV	postoperative nausea and vomiting
POP	pelvic organ prolapse; persistent occiput posterior; progestin-only pill
pop	popliteal
PORP	partial ossicular replacement prosthesis
POS	point of service; problem-oriented system
pos	positive

poss	possible
post	after; posterior
post-op	postoperative
POTx	proof of treatment
PP	placenta previa; postpartum; postprandial; pulse pressure; pulsus paradoxus
PPA	phenylpyruvic acid; preferred provider arrangement; primary progressive aphasia
PPB	positive pressure breathing
ppb	parts per billion
PPBG	postprandial blood glucose
PPBS	postprandial blood sugar
PPD	packs per day; postpartum depression; purified protein derivative
P&PD	percussion and postural drainage
PPE	personal protective equipment
PPF	plasma protein fraction; posterior pharyngeal flap
PPG	postprandial glucose
PPH	postpartum hemorrhage; primary pulmonary hypertension; procedure for prolapse and hemorrhoids
PPHN	persistent pulmonary hypertension of the newborn
PPHx	previous psychiatric history
PPI	patient package insert; proton pump inhibitor
PPIP	Put Prevention Into Practice
PPM	permanent pacemaker; planned preventive maintenance
ppm	parts per million

PPMA	postpoliomyelitis muscular atrophy
PPN	peripheral parenteral nutrition
PPO	preferred provider organization
PPR	potentially preventable readmission
PPROM	preterm premature rupture of membranes
PPS	postpartum sterilization
PPT	partial prothrombin time; plasma preparation tube
PPTC	Pediatric Preclinical Testing Consortium
PPTCT	Prevention of Parent to Child Transmission
PPTL	postpartum tubal ligation
PPTP	Pediatric Preclinical Testing Program
PPV	pneumococcal polysaccharide vaccine; positive predictive value; positive pressure ventilation
PPW	pre-pregnancy weight
PQRST	provocation/palliation, quality/quantity, region/radiation, severity scale, timing
PR	per rectum; proctology; Proctologist; prothrombin ratio; pulmonic regurgitation; pulse rate
P&R	pulse and respiration
PR3	proteinase 3
PRA	panel reactive antibody; plasma renin activity
PRB	partial rebreather
PRBC	packed red blood cell
PRE	progressive resistance exercise
PREA	Pediatric Research Equity Act
preg	pregnant/pregnancy
PREM	Patient-reported experience measure

pre-op	preoperative
PrEP	pre-exposure prophylaxis
prep	prepare/preparation
PRES	posterior reversible encephalopathy syndrome
prev	preventive/prevention; previous
PRF	Provider Relief Fund
PRG	progesterone
PRH	pregnancy-related hypertension; prolactin-releasing hormone
primip	primipara
PRIND	prolonged reversible ischemic neurologic deficit
PRK	photorefractive keratectomy
PRL	prolactin
prn	as needed (pro re nata)
PRO	Peer Review Organization; Professional Review Organization
pro time, PT	prothrombin time
prob	probable
prog, Px	prognosis
PROM	partial range of motion; passive range of motion; patient-reported outcome measure; prelabor rupture of membranes; premature rupture of membranes
pron	pronate/pronation
prosth	prosthesis
prox	proximal
PRP	panretinal photocoagulation; platelet-rich plasma; progressive rubella panencephalitis
PrP	prion protein
PRRB	Provider Reimbursement Review Board

PRRT	Pediatric Rapid Response Team
PRSP	penicillin-resistant Streptococcus pneumoniae
PRT	progressive resistance training
PRTF	psychiatric residential treatment facility
PRV	polycythemia rubra vera
PRVC	pressure-regulated volume control
PS	pressure support; pulmonary stenosis
PSA	prostate-specific antigen; public service announcement
PsA, PA	psoriatic arthritis
PSBO	partial small bowel obstruction
PSC	primary sclerosing cholangitis
PSCT	peripheral stem cell transplant
PSDA	Patient Self-Determination Act
PSE	portal systemic encephalopathy
PSG	polysomnogram; polysomnography
PSGN	poststreptococcal glomerulonephritis
PSH	paroxysmal sympathetic hyperactivity; past surgical history; psychosocial history
PSI	Patient Safety Indicator; pneumonia severity index; pounds per square inch
PSIS	posterior superior iliac spine
PSN	provider sponsored network
PSO	provider sponsored organization
PSP	phenolsulfonphthalein
PSS	progressive systemic sclerosis
PST	preoperative systemic therapy; primary systemic therapy
PSV	pressure support ventilation

PSVT	paroxysmal supraventricular tachycardia
psy, psych	psychiatry; psychology
PsyD	Doctor of Psychology
PT	part time; physical therapy; Physical Therapist; preferred term; prothrombin time
pt	patient
PTA	peritonsillar abscess; percutaneous transluminal angioplasty; Physical Therapist Assistant; post-traumatic amnesia; prior to admission; prior to arrival; pure tone audiometry
PTB	pulmonary tuberculosis
PTC	papillary thyroid cancer; percutaneous transhepatic cholangiogram; percutaneous transhepatic cholangiography
PTCA	percutaneous transluminal coronary angioplasty
PTD	preterm delivery
PTE	pulmonary thromboembolism
PTFE	polytetrafluorethylene
PTH	parathormone; parathyroid hormone
PTHC, PTC	percutaneous transhepatic cholangiography
PTK	phototherapeutic keratectomy
PTL	preterm labor
PTSD	post-traumatic stress disorder
PTSS	post-traumatic stress syndrome
PTT	partial thromboplastin time
PTTD	posterior tibial tendonitis dysfunction
PTX, PNX	pneumothorax
PU	palindromic unit; peptic ulcer
p/u	pick up
PUBS	percutaneous umbilical blood sampling

PUD	peptic ulcer disease
PUFA	polyunsaturated fatty acid
PUI	patient under investigation
pul, pulm	pulmonary
pulv	powder (pulvis)
PUMS	Public Use Microdata Sample
PUO	pyrexia of unknown origin
PUSH	Pressure Ulcer Scale for Healing
PUVA	psoralen plus ultraviolet A
PV	polycythemia vera; portal vein; pulmonary valve; vaginal/vaginally (per vaginam)
PVC	polyvinyl chloride; premature ventricular contraction
PVD	peripheral vascular disease; posterior vitreous detachment
PVFS	post-viral fatigue syndrome
PVI	peripheral vascular insufficiency; pulmonary vein isolation
PVOD	pulmonary veno-occlusive disease
PVR	peripheral vascular resistance; pulmonary vascular resistance; post-void residual
PVRI	pulmonary vascular resistance index
PVS	persistent vegetative state; Plummer-Vinson syndrome; pulmonary valve stenosis
PVT	paroxysmal ventricular tachycardia
PVW	posterior vaginal wall
PWA	person with AIDS
PWB	partial weight bearing
PWD	pink, warm, dry
pwdr, pdr	powder

PWP	pulmonary wedge pressure
PX, PE, PEX	physical examination
Px, prog	prognosis
PYLL	potential years of life lost
q	each; every (quaque)
q1h, q2h, etc.	every 1 hour, every 2 hours, etc.
QA	quality assurance
QALY	quality-adjusted life year
qAM, qam	every day before noon (quaque ante meridiem)
QAPI	Quality Assurance and Performance Improvement
Qb	blood flow
QC	quality control
QCT	quantitative computed tomography
qd*	once a day*; every day (quaque die)*
qh	each hour; every hour (quaque hora)
QHP	qualified health plan; qualified healthcare professional
qhs*	every night at bedtime (quaque hora somni)*
QI	quality improvement
qid	four times a day (quater in die)
QIDS	Quick Inventory of Depressive Symptomatology
QIS	qualified in specialty
ql	as much as desired (quantum libet)
QM	quality management
qm	every morning (quaque mane)
QMP	qualified medical practitioner
qn*	every night (quaque nocte)*
QNS	quantity not sufficient

qod*	every other day (quaque altera die)*
qoh	every other hour (quaque altera hora)
QOL	quality of life
QOM	quality of motion; quality of movement
qon	every other night (quaque altera nocte)
QOR	quality of recovery
qp	as much as desired (quantum placeat)
qPCR	quantitative polymerase chain reaction
qPM, qpm	every day after noon (quaque post meridiem)
QR	quality review
QRNG	quinolone-resistant Neisseria gonorrhoeae
qs	sufficient quantity (quantum sufficit)
qs ad	sufficient quantity to make (quantum sufficit ad)
Qs/Qt	shunt fraction
Qt, CO	cardiac output
qt	quart
QTD	quarter-to-date
qty, quant	quantity
quad	quadrant; quadricep; quadriplegic
qv	as much as desired (quantum vis); see also (quod vide)
qwk, qw	every week
RA	refractory anemia; rheumatoid arthritis; right arm; right atrium
RAA	relative antitumor activity; renal artery aneurysm; right atrial appendage
RAAS	renin-angiotensin-aldosterone system
rAb	recombinant antibody
RACE	rescue, alarm, confine, extinguish/evacuate

RAD	radiation absorbed dose; reactive airway disease; reactive attachment disorder; reflex anal dilation; right axis deviation; right anterior descending (artery)
rad	radial; radical
RAE	right atrial enlargement
RAFB	right anterior fascicular block
RAH	right atrial hypertrophy
RAHA	rheumatoid arthritis hemagglutination assay
RAI	radioactive iodine; Resident Assessment Instrument
RAIU	radioactive iodine uptake
RALH	robot-assisted laparoscopic hysterectomy
RAM	rapid alternating movement
RANA	rheumatoid arthritis nuclear antigen
RAO	right anterior oblique
RAP	Resident Assessment Protocol; right atrial pressure
RAPD	relative afferent pupillary defect
RAS	renal artery stenosis; reticular activating system
RAST	radioallergosorbent test
r/b	referred by; relieved by
RBBB	right bundle branch block
RBC	red blood cell; red blood count
RBE	relative biological effectiveness
RBLM	recurrent benign lymphocytic meningitis
RBP	resting blood pressure; retinol-binding protein
RBV	readback verification
RCA	right coronary artery

RCC	renal cell carcinoma
RCF	residential care facility; right cubital fossa
RCIS	Registered Cardiovascular Invasive Specialist
RCL	radial collateral ligament
RCM	restrictive cardiomyopathy; right costal margin
RCP	Respiratory Care Practitioner
RCR	replication competent retrovirus; rotator cuff repair
RCS	Registered Cardiac Sonographer
RCT	randomized clinical trial; randomized controlled trial; rotator cuff tear
RCU	respiratory care unit
RCX	ramus circumflex artery
RD	radial deviation; Registered Dietician; Raynaud disease; respiratory disease; respiratory distress; retinal detachment; right deltoid
R&D	research and development
RDA	recommended daily allowance; recommended dietary allowance
RDH	Registered Dental Hygienist
RDI	reference daily intake; recommended daily intake; recommended dietary intake; respiratory distress index; respiratory disturbance index
RDMS	Registered Diagnostic Medical Sonographer
RDP	random donor platelet
RDS	respiratory distress syndrome
RDT	rapid diagnostic test; rising dose tolerance
RDU	rheumatic disease unit
RDW	red cell distribution width

RE	reconditioning exercise; rectal examination; right eye
ReA	reactive arthritis
reb	rebound
REBT	rational emotive behavioral therapy
rec	recommend
REE	resting energy expenditure
ref	refer/referral; refused
refl	reflex
reg	regular
rehab	rehabilitation
REI	reproductive endocrinology and infertility
rel	related; relative
REM	rapid eye movement
rem	remove
REMS	rapid eye movement sleep; Risk Evaluation and Mitigation Strategy
reps	repetitions
RES	reticuloendothelial system
resc	rescue
resid	residual
resp	respiration/respiratory; response
resus	resuscitation
RET	rational emotive therapy
retic	reticulocyte
retro	retrograde
rev	reverse; review; revision; revolution
RF	retroflexed/retroflexion; rheumatic fever; rheumatoid factor; risk factor

r/f	refill
RFA	radiofrequency ablation; right femoral artery; right forearm; right frontoanterior
RFFF	radial forearm free flap
RFLP	restriction fragment length polymorphism
RFP	right frontoposterior
RFT	renal function test; right frontotransverse
RGA	retrograde amnesia
RGM	rubs, gallops, murmurs
RH	right hand
Rh	Rhesus (factor)
RHC	right heart catheterization; rural health clinic
RHD	rheumatic heart disease
RHF	right heart failure
RHIA	Registered Health Information Administrator
RHIO	Regional Health Information Organization
RHR	resting heart rate
RIA	radioimmunoassay
RIBA	recombinant immunoblot assay
RICE	rest, ice, compression, elevation
RID	radial immunodiffusion
RIG	rabies immune globulin
RIH	right inguinal hernia
RIMA	reversible inhibitor of monoamine oxidase A; right internal mammary artery
RIND	reversible ischemic neurologic deficit
RK	radial keratotomy
RL*	right lateral; right leg*; right lung*
R/L, R-L	right to left

RLAS	Rancho Los Amigos Scale
RLE	right lower extremity
RLL	right lower lobe
RLN	recurrent laryngeal nerve
RLQ	right lower quadrant
RLS	restless leg syndrome
RLSB	right lower sternal border
RM	respiratory movement
RMA	refused medical assistance; right mentoanterior
RMCA	right main coronary artery
RML	right mediolateral; right middle lobe
RMS	rhabdomyosarcoma
RMSF	Rocky Mountain spotted fever
RMT	retromolar trigone; right mentotransverse
RN	Registered Nurse
RNA	ribonucleic acid
RN-C	Registered Nurse-Certified
RNFA	Registered Nurse First Assistant
RNP	ribonucleoprotein
RNV, RVG	radionuclide ventriculogram; radionuclide ventriculography
r/o	rule out
ROA	right occiput anterior
ROI	release of information
ROM	range of motion; recurrent otitis media; rupture of membranes
ROP	retinopathy of prematurity; right occiput posterior
ROS	review of symptoms; review of systems

ROSC	return of spontaneous circulation
ROT	right occiput transverse
rot	rotation
RP	Raynaud's phenomenon; retinitis pigmentosa
RPE	rate of perceived exertion
RPF	renal plasma flow
RPG	retrograde pyelogram; retrograde pyelography
RPGN	rapidly progressive glomerulonephritis
RPh	Registered Pharmacist
RPLND	retroperitoneal lymph node dissection
RPM	revolutions per minute
RPO	right posterior oblique
RPP	rate pressure product; renal perfusion pressure
RPR	rapid plasma reagin
RPT	Registered Physical Therapist
RQ	respiratory quotient
RR	recovery room; relative risk; respiratory rate
RRA	Registered Record Administrator
RRMS	relapsing-remitting multiple sclerosis
rRNA	ribosomal RNA
RRP	radical retropubic prostatectomy; recurrent respiratory papillomatosis
RRR	regular rate and rhythm
RRT	Rapid Response Team; Registered Respiratory Therapist
RS*	Reiter's syndrome*; Reye's syndrome*
r/s	reschedule
RS3PE	remitting seronegative symmetrical synovitis with pitting edema

RSA	right sacrum anterior
RSB	right sternal border
RSBI	rapid shallow breathing index
RSC	right subclavian
RSD	reflex sympathetic dystrophy
RSI	rapid sequence induction; repetitive strain injury; repetitive stress injury
RSO	right salpingo-oophorectomy
RSP	right sacrum posterior
RSR	regular sinus rhythm
RST	right sacrum transverse
RT	radiation therapy; radiotherapy; respiratory therapy; Radiologic Technologist; Registered Therapist; Respiratory Therapist; reverse transcriptase
rt	right
r/t	related to
RTA	renal tubular acidosis
RTC	return to clinic
RTF	residential treatment facility
RTI	respiratory tract infection; reverse transcriptase inhibitor
RT-PCR	reverse transcriptase-polymerase chain reaction
RTS	Revised Trauma Score
RTW	return to work
RTx, RT, XRT	radiation therapy; radiotherapy
RUA	right upper arm
RUD	right uterine displacement
RUE	right upper extremity

RUG	Resource Utilization Group; retrograde urethrogram; retrograde urethrography
RUL	right upper lobe
RUO	research use only
rupt	rupture
RUQ	right upper quadrant
RUTI	recurrent urinary tract infection
RV	residual volume; retroverted; retroviral; return visit; right ventricle; rotavirus
RVA	rabies vaccine adsorbed; right ventricular aneurysm
RVAD	right ventricular assist device
RVC	responds to verbal commands
RVCT	report of verified case of tuberculosis
RVE	right ventricular enlargement
RVEDP	right ventricular end-diastolic pressure
RVEF	right ventricular ejection fraction
RVET	right ventricular ejection time
RVF	rectovaginal fistula; right ventricular failure; right ventricular function
RVG, RNV	radionuclide ventriculogram; radionuclide ventriculography
RVH	right ventricular hypertrophy
RVPW	right ventricular posterior wall
RVR	rapid ventricular response
RVS	rectovaginal septum; Registered Vascular Specialist
RVSP	right ventricular systolic pressure
RVSV	right ventricular stroke volume
RVT	renal vein thrombosis

RVVC	recurrent vulvovaginal candidiasis
R&W	recreation and welfare
Rx	drug; medication; medicine; prescription; therapy
rxn	reaction
RXT	right exotropia
$\overline{s}$	without (sine)
S1, S2, etc.	heart sound (first, second, etc.); sacral vertebrae (first, second, etc.)
SA*	salicylic acid; sexual assault; sinoatrial; sinus arrhythmia; stomach ache; sustained action; suicide alert*; suicide attempt*
sa	use your judgment (secundum artem)
SAA	synthetic amino acid
SAAG	serum-ascites albumin gradient
SAARD	slow-acting antirheumatic drug
SAB	spontaneous abortion
SAC	short arm cast
SAD*	single ascending dose; seasonal affective disorder*; social anxiety disorder*
SAE	serious adverse event
SAH	subarachnoid hemorrhage
SALT, SLT	speech and language therapy
SAM	systolic anterior motion
SAN	sinoatrial node
SANE	Sexual Assault Nurse Examiner
SaO_2, O_2 sat	oxygen saturation
SAR	seasonal allergic rhinitis
SARS	severe acute respiratory syndrome

SAS	Symptom Assessment Scale
sat	saturate/saturation
SB	sinus bradycardia; small bowel
SBAR	situation, background, assessment, recommendation
SBC	Summary of Benefits and Coverage
SBE	self breast examination; subacute bacterial endocarditis
SBFT	small bowel follow through
SBGM	self blood glucose monitoring
SBMA	spinal and bulbar muscular atrophy
SBO	small bowel obstruction
SBP	spontaneous bacterial peritonitis; systolic blood pressure
SBR	serum bilirubin
SBRT	stereotactic body radiation therapy
SBS	shaken baby syndrome; short bowel syndrome; small bowel series
SC*	spinal cord; subcutaneous*
SCA	sickle cell anemia; spinocerebellar ataxia
SCAD	schizoaffective disorder
SCADD	short-chain acyl-CoA dehydrogenase deficiency
SCAT	sheep cell agglutination test
SCC	Skilled Care Coordinator; squamous cell carcinoma
SCD	sequential compression device; sickle cell disease; sudden cardiac death
SCFE	slipped capital femoral epiphysis
SCHIP	State Children's Health Insurance Program
SCI	spinal cord injury

sci	science
SCID	severe combined immunodeficiency
SCIWORA	spinal cord injury without radiographic abnormality
SCL	soft contact lens
SCLC	small cell lung cancer
SCLE	subacute cutaneous lupus erythematosus
SCM	sternocleidomastoid
SCN	special care nursery
scope	endoscope; microscope
SCr	serum creatinine
SCT	sacrococcygeal teratoma; stem cell transplant; sickle cell trait; Specialist in Cytotechnology
SCTAT	sex cord tumors with annular tubules
SCU	special care unit
SCZ	schizophrenia
SD	skin dose; standard deviation; subdermal
SDAT	senile dementia of the Alzheimer's type
SDH	subdural hematoma
SDP	single donor platelet
SDSU	same-day surgery unit
SDT	speech detection threshold
sDTI	suspected deep tissue injury
SE	side effect; substantial equivalence; standard error
sec	second
SED	skin erythema dose
sed rate	sedimentation rate
SEE	Syphilis Elimination Effort

SEER	Surveillance, Epidemiology, and End Results
seg	segment
SEM	systolic ejection murmur
SEMI	subendocardial myocardial infarction
semih	half an hour (sēmihōra)
sens	sensation; sensitive/sensitivity; sensory
SEP	somatosensory evoked potential; special enrollment period
sep	separate
seq	sequence
SERM	selective estrogen receptor modulator
SERT	serotonin transporter
SES	socioeconomic status
SF	safety factor; serum ferritin; sugar free; synovial fluid
SFA	serum folic acid; superficial femoral artery
sFe, SI	serum iron
SFV	superficial femoral vein
SG	salivary gland; serum glucose; skin graft; specific gravity; suicide gesture
SGA	small for gestational age
SGB	stellate ganglion block
SGC	Swan-Ganz catheter
SGOT	serum glutamic oxaloacetic transaminase
SGPT	serum glutamic pyruvic transaminase
SGS	subglottic stenosis
SH	serum hepatitis; social history; surgical history
SHBG	sex hormone-binding globulin
SHFFT	Surgical Hip and Femur Fracture Treatment

SHIP	State Health Innovation Plan
SHOP	Small Business Health Options Program
SHP, SHPT	secondary hyperparathyroidism
SI	International System of Units (Système International); sacroiliac; serious incident; serum iron; stroke index; suicidal ideation
SIA	strip immunoblot assay
SIADH	syndrome of inappropriate antidiuretic hormone
SIB	self-injurious behavior
sib	sibling
SIBO	small intestinal bacterial overgrowth
SICC	Skilled Inpatient Care Coordinator
SICU	surgical intensive care unit
SIDS	sudden infant death syndrome
SIE	serious infection event; severe ischemic event; stroke-in-evolution
sig	label (signa); signal; signature
SIHD	stable ischemic heart disease
SIL	squamous intraepithelial lesion
sim	similar; simulate
SIMD	substance-induced mood disorder
simul	simultaneously
SIMV	synchronized intermittent mandatory ventilation
SIP	sterilization-in-place
SIRES	stabilize, identify toxin, reverse effect, eliminate toxin, support
SIRI	serious incident requiring investigation
SIRS	systemic inflammatory response syndrome

SIS, SHG	saline infusion sonohysterogram; saline infusion sonohysterography
SIT	Slosson Intelligence Test; stress inoculation training
SIVP	slow intravenous push
SIW	self-inflicted wound
SJS*	Schwartz-Jampel syndrome*; Stevens-Johnson syndrome*
SjS, SS	Sjögren's syndrome
SK	seborrheic keratosis
skel	skeletal
SL	saline lock; sublingual
sl	slight/slightly
SLB	short leg brace
SLD	specific learning disability
SLE	Saint Louis encephalitis; slit-lamp examination; systemic lupus erythematosus
SLEV	Saint Louis encephalitis virus
SLL	small lymphocytic lymphoma
SLN	sentinel lymph node
SLNB	sentinel lymph node biopsy
SLP	speech-language pathology; Speech-Language Pathologist
SLR	straight leg raise
SLT, SALT	speech and language therapy
SM	skeletal muscle; synovial membrane; submucosal
sm	small
SMA	smooth muscle antibody; spinal muscular atrophy; superior mesenteric artery

SMBG	self-monitoring of blood glucose
SMD	senile macular degeneration
SMG	submandibular gland
SMN	Statement of Medical Necessity
SMR	sleeping metabolic rate; standardized mortality ratio; submucous resection
SMT	spinal manipulative therapy
SMV	superior mesenteric vein
SN	sentinel node; skilled nursing; Student Nurse
SNB	sentinel node biopsy
SNF	skilled nursing facility
SNHL	sensorineural hearing loss
SNOMED	Systematized Nomenclature of Medicine
SNP	single nucleotide polymorphism; Special Needs Plan
SNRI	serotonin and norepinephrine reuptake inhibitor
snRNP	small nuclear ribonucleoprotein
SNS	supplemental nursing system; sympathetic nervous system
SNV	Sin Nombre virus
SO	salpingo-oophorectomy
SOA	swelling of ankle
SOAP	subjective, objective, assessment, plan
SOAPIER	subjective, objective, assessment, plan, intervention, evaluation, response
SOB	shortness of breath; side of bed
SOBOE	shortness of breath on exertion
SOC	standard of care
SOI	severity of illness

SOL	space-occupying lesion
sol	solute/solution; soluble
SOM	serous otitis media
SOMI	sternal occipital mandibular immobilizer
SON	superior ovarian nerve; supraorbital nerve
sono	sonogram; sonography
SOP	standard operating procedure
SOS	if necessary (si opus sit); sinusoidal obstruction syndrome; distress signal
SOT	sacro-occipital technique; sensory organization test; solid organ transplant
SP	specialty pharmacy; suprapubic
sp	space; species; spine/spinal
s/p	status post
SpA	spondyloarthropathy
sPAP	systolic pulmonary artery pressure
SPC	specialist palliative care; suprapubic catheter
SPE	State Partnership Exchange; streptococcal pyrogenic exotoxin
spec	specification; specimen
SPECT	single photon emission computed tomography
SPEP	serum protein electrophoresis
SPF	sun protection factor
SPLATT	symptoms, previous falls, location, activity, time, trauma
SpO_2	peripheral capillary oxygen saturation
spon, spont	spontaneous
SPP	specialty pharmacy provider; suprapubic prostatectomy

spp	several species (species pluralis)
SPROM	spontaneous preterm rupture of membranes
SQ, Sub-Q, SC*	subcutaneous*
sq	squamous
SR	sinus rhythm; slow release; sustained release
SRD	single rising dose
SRI	serotonin reuptake inhibitor
sRNA	soluble RNA
SROM, SRM	spontaneous rupture of membranes
SRS	sex reassignment surgery; stereotactic radiosurgery
SRT	speech recognition threshold; stereotactic radiation therapy
SS	Sjögren's syndrome; Social Services
$\overline{s}\,\overline{s}$ *	half (sēmis)*
S/S, S/Sx	signs/symptoms
SSA	sessile serrated adenoma
SSC	secondary sexual characteristic
SSc	systemic sclerosis
SSDI	Social Security Disability Insurance
ssDNA	single-stranded DNA
SSE*	saline solution enema*; soap suds enema*; sterile speculum examination
SSEP, SEP	somatosensory evoked potential
SSI*	sliding scale insulin*; Supplemental Security Income; surgical site infection
SSKI	saturated solution of potassium iodide
SSN, SS#	Social Security number
SSNHL, SSHL	sudden sensorineural hearing loss

SSO	second surgical opinion
SSPE	subacute sclerosing panencephalitis
SSRI*	selective serotonin reuptake inhibitor*; sliding scale regular insulin*
ssRNA	single-stranded RNA
SSS	sick sinus syndrome
SSSI	skin and skin-structure infection
SSSS	staphylococcal scalded skin syndrome
ST	sinus tachycardia; speech therapy; Speech Therapist
st	let it stand (stet); stomach; straight
staph	staphylococcus
START	simple triage and rapid treatment
stat	immediately (statim)
STD	sexually transmitted disease; short-term disability
STEL	short-term exposure limit
STEMI	ST-elevation myocardial infarction
ster	sterile
STH	somatotropic hormone
STI	sexually transmitted infection; soft tissue injury
stim	stimulate/stimulation
STM	short-term memory
STN	subthalamic nucleus
STNR	symmetrical tonic neck reflex
strep	streptococcus
STRIVE	Staff Time and Resource Intensity Verification
STS	serological test for syphilis; soft tissue sarcoma
STSG	split-thickness skin graft

STV	short-term variability
SUA	serum uric acid
Sub.Q, SQ, SC*	subcutaneous*
suc	sucrose
SUD	single-use device; substance use disorder; sudden unexpected death
SUDEP	sudden unexpected death in epilepsy
SUI	stress urinary incontinence
SUID	sudden unexpected infant death
sup, supr	superior
supf	superficial
supp	suppository
surg	surgery/surgical
SUS	scanning ultrasound
susp	suspension
sut	suture
SUV	standardized uptake value
SV	saphenous vein; seminal vesicle; stroke volume; supraventricular
SVC	seminal vesicle cyst; superior vena cava
SVD	spontaneous vaginal delivery
SVE	sterile vaginal examination
SVG	saphenous vein graft
SVI	stroke volume index
SVN	small volume nebulizer
SVR	sustained virologic response; systemic vascular resistance
SVRI	systemic vascular resistance index
SVT	supraventricular tachycardia

SW	social work; social worker; stab wound
SWD	short wave diathermy
SWI	surgical wound infection
SWL	shockwave lithotripsy
SWS	Sturge-Weber syndrome
Sx	surgery; symptom
SXR	skull x-ray
sym, symm	symmetrical
syn, synth	synthetic
syph	syphilis
syr	syringe; syrup
sys	system
syst	systolic
sz	seizure
T, tbs, tbsp	tablespoon
t, tsp	teaspoon
T1, T2, etc.	thoracic vertebrae (first, second, etc.)
T3, T_3	triiodothyronine
T4, T_4	tetraiodothyronine; thyroxine
TA	temporal arteritis; toxin-antitoxin; tentative approval
T&A	tonsillectomy and adenoidectomy
TAA	thoracic aortic aneurysm
TAB	therapeutic abortion; threatened abortion; total androgen block
tab	tablet
tachy	tachycardia
TAD	take as directed
TAF	Triage Assessment Form

TAH	total abdominal hysterectomy; total artificial heart; transfusion-associated hepatitis
TAM	total active motion
TANF	Temporary Assistance for Needy Families
TAP	trypsinogen activation peptide
TAPVR	total anomalous pulmonary venous return
TAR	total ankle replacement
TAROM	total active range of motion
TAT	tetanus antitoxin; Thematic Apperception Test; turnaround time
TAVI	transcatheter aortic valve implantation
TAVR	transcatheter aortic valve replacement
TB	total bilirubin; tracheobronchial; tuberculosis; tubercle bacillus
TBA*	to be admitted*; to be announced*
TBB, TBBx	transbronchial biopsy
TBBMC	total body bone mineral content
TBBMD	total body bone mineral density
TBG	thyroid-binding globulin; thyroxine-binding globulin
TBI	total body irradiation; traumatic brain injury
TBSA	total body surface area
TBT	tracheobronchial tree
TBW	total body water; total body weight
TC	tactile cue; therapeutic community; thoracic cavity; total cholesterol; trauma center
T&C, T&X	type and cross; type and crossmatch
t/c	to consider
TCA	trichloroacetic acid; tricyclic antidepressant

TCC	transitional cell cancer; transitional cell carcinoma
TCD	transcranial Doppler
TCDB	turn, cough, deep breath
TCM	traditional Chinese medicine
TCOM	transcutaneous oxygen measurement
TCP	thrombocytopenia
TCPI	Transforming Clinical Practice Initiative
TCPL	time-cycled, pressure-limited
TCT	thrombin clotting time
TCU	transitional care unit
TD	tardive dyskinesia; transdermal
Tdap	tetanus, diphtheria, pertussis (vaccine)
TDD	telecommunication device for the deaf; total daily dose; transdermal drug delivery
TDF	testis-determining factor
TDM	therapeutic drug monitoring
TdP	torsades de pointes
tds	three times a day (ter die sumendum)
TdT	terminal deoxynucleotidyl transferase
TE	therapeutic education; therapeutic equivalence; thromboembolism; toxoplasmic encephalitis
TEB	thoracic electrical bioimpedance
TEC	transient erythroblastopenia of childhood
TED	thromboembolic deterrent; transesophageal Doppler
TEE	total energy expenditure; transesophageal echocardiogram; transesophageal echocardiography
TEF	tracheoesophageal fistula

TEM	transmission electron microscopy
temp	temperature
TEN	toxic epidermal necrolysis
TEP	tracheoesophageal puncture
TET	treadmill exercise test
tet	tetanus
TF	tube feeding
TFR	total fluid removal; transdermal fluid removal; tumor volume to fetal weight ratio
TFS	testicular feminization syndrome
TFT	thyroid function test
TG, TRG, trig	triglyceride
Tg	thyroglobulin
TGA	transient global amnesia; transposition of the great arteries
TGF	transforming growth factor
T&H	type and hold
THA	total hip arthroplasty
THC	tetrahydrocannabinol
ther	therapeutic; therapy
THR	target heart rate; total hip replacement
TI	terminal ileum; thoracic inlet
TIA	transient ischemic attack
tib	tibia/tibial
TIBC	total iron-binding capacity
TICU*	transplant intensive care unit*; trauma intensive care unit*
tid	three times a day (ter in die)
TIG	tetanus immune globulin

TIH	tumor-induced hypercalcemia
TIN	tubulointerstitial nephritis
tin	three times a night (ter in nocte)
tinc	tincture
TIPS	transjugular intrahepatic portosystemic shunt
tiw*	three times a week*
TJA	total joint arthroplasty
TJC	The Joint Commission
TKA	total knee arthroplasty; trochanter-knee-ankle
TKE	terminal knee extension
TKO	to keep open
TKR	total knee replacement
TL	total laryngectomy; translingual; tubal ligation
TLC	total lymphocyte count; total lung capacity; triple-lumen catheter; thin layer chromatogram; thin layer chromatography; therapeutic lifestyle change
TLH	total laparoscopic hysterectomy
TLI	total lymphoid irradiation
TLR	tonic labyrinthine reflex
TLS	tumor lysis syndrome
TLSO	thoracic lumbar sacral orthosis
TM	temporomandibular; tympanic membrane
TMD	temporomandibular disorder
TME	total mesorectal excision; toxic metabolic encephalopathy
TMJ	temporomandibular joint
TMR	transmyocardial revascularization
TMT	treadmill test

TN	trigeminal neuralgia
TNA	total nail avulsion
TNBC	triple-negative breast cancer
TNF	tumor necrosis factor
TNM	tumor, node, metastasis
TNS	transcutaneous nerve stimulation; trigeminal nerve stimulation
TNTC	too numerous to count
TO	telephone order
TOA	tubo-ovarian abscess
TOC	test of cure
TOD	target organ damage
TOF	tetralogy of Fallot
tol	tolerate/tolerance
TOLAC	trial of labor after cesarean
TOP	termination of pregnancy
top	topical/topically
tOPV	trivalent oral poliovirus vaccine
TORB	telephone order read back
TORCH	toxoplasmosis, other (HIV, syphilis, etc.), rubella, cytomegalovirus, herpes simplex
TORP	total ossicular replacement prosthesis
TOS	thoracic outlet syndrome
TOT	transobturator tape
tox	toxic/toxicity; toxicology; Toxicologist
toxo	toxoplasmosis
TP	total protein
TPA	total parenteral alimentation
tPA	tissue plasminogen activator

TPE	therapeutic plasma exchange; total plasma exchange
TPI	Treponema pallidum immobilization; trigger point injection
TPN	total parenteral nutrition
TPO	thyroid peroxidase
TPPA	Treponema pallidum particle agglutination
TPR	temperature, pulse, respiration; total peripheral resistance
TR	therapeutic recreation; timed release; tricuspid regurgitation
tr	trace; treatment
TRAb	thyrotropin receptor antibody
trach	trachea/tracheal; tracheostomy; tracheotomy
TRALI	transfusion-related acute lung injury
TRAM	transverse rectus abdominis myocutaneous
trans	transverse
TRAP	tartrate-resistant acid phosphatase; tremor, rigidity, akinesia, postural instability
TRBF	total renal blood flow
Treg	regulatory T cell
TRF, xfer	transfer
TRH	thyroid-releasing hormone; thyrotropin-releasing hormone
trich	trichomoniasis
trig, TRG, TG	triglyceride
trit	triturate
TRM	treatment-related mortality
tRNA	transfer RNA
TrOOP	true out of pocket

TRT	testosterone replacement therapy
TRUS	transrectal ultrasound
TS*	Tourette syndrome*; Turner syndrome*; tricuspid stenosis
T&S	type and screen
TSD	time since death
TSE	testicular self-examination; transmissible spongiform encephalopathy
TSF	triceps skinfold
TSH	thoughts of self-harm; thyroid-stimulating hormone
TSI	thyroid-stimulating immunoglobulin
tsp, t	teaspoon
T-spine	thoracic spine
TSR	total sodium removal
TSS	toxic shock syndrome
TST	tuberculin skin test
TT	tetanus toxoid; thrombin time; thrombolytic therapy; total thyroidectomy
TTE	transthoracic echocardiogram; transthoracic echocardiography
tTG	tissue transglutaminase
TTN	transient tachypnea of the newborn
TTP	thrombotic thrombocytopenic purpura; tenderness to palpation
TTR	transthyretin
TTS	thrombosis with thrombocytopenia syndrome; transdermal therapeutic system
TTT	tilt table test
TTTS	twin-to-twin transfusion syndrome

TTY	teletypewriter; text telephone
TU	tuberculin unit
TUBA	transumbilical breast augmentation
TUI	transurethral incision
TUIP	transurethral incision of prostate
TUMA	transurethral microwave antenna
TUMT	transurethral microwave therapy; transurethral microwave thermotherapy
TUNA	transurethral needle ablation
TUR	transurethral resection
TURBT	transurethral resection of bladder tumor
TURP	transurethral resection of prostate
TV	tidal volume; total volume; tricuspid valve
TVH	total vaginal hysterectomy
TVR	tricuspid valve replacement
TVT	tension-free vaginal tape
TVU, TVUS	transvaginal ultrasound
tw, biw	twice a week
TWOC	trial without catheter
Tx*	therapy*; traction*; transplant*; treatment*
T&X, T&C	type and cross; type and crossmatch
UA	unstable angina; uric acid; urinalysis
UAC	umbilical artery catheter; urinary albumin concentration
UAE	uterine artery embolization
UAO	upper airway obstruction
UAP	unlicensed assistive personnel; unstable angina pectoris
UB	upper body

UBD	universal blood donor
UBT	urea breath test
UC	ulcerative colitis; umbilical cord; urothelial carcinoma; uterine contraction
UCB	umbilical cord blood
UCC	uncompensated care; urgent care center
UCD, UCHD	usual childhood diseases
UCDS	Uniform Clinical Data Set
UCL	ulnar collateral ligament
UCR	usual, customary, reasonable
UCTD	undifferentiated connective tissue disease
UCx	urine culture
UD	ulnar deviation; unit dose
ud, ut dict	as directed (ut dictum)
UDS	undifferentiated sarcoma; urine drug screen; urodynamic study
UDT	urine drug test
UE	upper extremity
U&E	urea and electrolytes
UES	upper esophageal sphincter
UF	ultrafiltration; uroflowmetry
UFC	urinary free cortisol
UFE	uterine fibroid embolization
UFR	ultrafiltration rate
UG	urogenital
UGI	upper gastrointestinal
UHDDS	Uniform Hospital Discharge Data Set
UIP	usual interstitial pneumonia
UIQ	upper inner quadrant

UL, UIL	upper intake level
U&L	upper and lower
ULN	upper limit of normal
ULQ	upper left quadrant
ult praes	last prescribed (ultimus praescriptus)
UM	utilization management
μm	micron
umb	umbilical/umbilicus
UMN	upper motor neuron
UN	unilateral nephrectomy; urea nitrogen
ung	ointment (unguentum)
unilat	unilateral
unk	unknown
UNOS	United Network for Organ Sharing
UO, UOP	urine output
u/o	under observation
UOA	upon our arrival
UOQ	upper outer quadrant
uPA	urokinase plasminogen activator
UPDRS	Unified Parkinson's Disease Rating Scale
UPEP	urine protein electrophoresis
UPJ	ureteropelvic junction
UPP	urethral pressure profile
UPPP	uvulopalatopharyngoplasty
UPT	urine pregnancy test
UQ	upper quadrant
UR	upper respiratory; utilization review
ur	urine
URA	unilateral renal agenesis

URD	upper respiratory disease
URI	upper respiratory infection
urol	urology; Urologist
URQ	upper right quadrant
URS	upper respiratory symptoms; ureteroscopy
URT	upper respiratory tract
URTI	upper respiratory tract infection
US	ultrasonic; ultrasound; ultrasonogram; ultrasonography
USAN	United States Adopted Name
USDHHS	United States Department of Health and Human Services
USN	ultrasonic nebulizer
USO	unilateral salpingo-oophorectomy
USOH	usual state of health
USP	United States Pharmacopeia
USPHS	United States Public Health Service
USR	unheated serum reagin
USS	ultrasound scan
UT	urinary tract
ut dict, ud	as directed (ut dictum)
UTD	up-to-date
UTI	urinary tract infection
UTUC	upper tract urothelial cancer
UTV	ultrasonic transmission velocity
UUN	urine urea nitrogen
UUS	upper uterine segment
UV	ultraviolet; umbilical vein; urine volume
UVA	ultraviolet A

UVB	ultraviolet B
UVC	ultraviolet C; umbilical venous catheter
UVGI	ultraviolet germicidal irradiation
UVJ	ureterovesical junction
V	volt
VA	visual acuity
VAB	venoarterial bypass
VAC	vacuum-assisted closure
vac, vax	vaccine/vaccination
VAD	vascular access device; venous access device; ventricular assist device
VAE	ventilator-associated event
VAERS	Vaccine Adverse Event Reporting System
vag	vagina/vaginal
VAIN	vaginal intraepithelial neoplasia
VAMP	vesicle-associated membrane protein
VAP	ventilator-associated pneumonia
var	variance/variation; variety
VAS	vibroacoustic stimulation; visual analog scale
vasc	vascular
VATS	video-assisted thoracoscopic surgery
VB	vaginal bleeding
VBAC	vaginal birth after cesarean
VBG	venous blood gas
VBP	value-based payment
VBW	vertical bitewing
VC	vena cava; vital capacity; vocal cord
VCE	video capsule endoscopy
VCF	vaginal contraceptive film

vCJD	variant Creutzfeldt-Jakob disease
VCP	vocal cord paralysis
VCT	venous clotting time
VCUG	voiding cystourethrogram; voiding cystourethrography
VD	vaginal delivery; venereal disease
vd	void
VDG	venereal disease, gonorrhea
VDRL	venereal disease research laboratory
VDS	venereal disease, syphilis
VE	vaccine efficacy; vaginal examination
VEB	ventricular ectopic beat
VEE	Venezuelan equine encephalitis
VEEV	Venezuelan equine encephalitis virus
VEF	ventricular ejection fraction
vent	ventilate/ventilator
VEP	visually evoked potential
VER	visually evoked response
vert	vertical
VF, V-fib	ventricular fibrillation
VFSS	videofluoroscopic swallow study
VG	ventrogluteal
VGE	viral gastroenteritis
VH	vaginal hysterectomy; viral hepatitis; visual hallucination
VHA	Voluntary Hospitals of America
VHD	valvular heart disease
VHDL	very high-density lipoprotein
via	by way of; through

VIG	vaccinia immune globulin
VIGIV	vaccinia immune globulin intravenous
VIN	vulvar intraepithelial neoplasia
VIP	vasoactive intestinal peptide; voluntary interruption of pregnancy
VIR	vascular and interventional radiology; Vascular and Interventional Radiologist
VIS	Vaccine Information Statement
vis	vision
vit	vitamin
VKA	vitamin K antagonist
VKC	vernal keratoconjunctivitis
VL	vastus lateralis; viral load
VLBW	very low birth weight
VLCAD	very long-chain acyl-CoA dehydrogenase deficiency
VLDL	very low-density lipoprotein
VM	venous malformation
VMA	vanillylmandelic acid
VNPI	Van Nuys Prognostic Index
VO	verbal order; voice order
VOC	vaso-occlusive crisis
VOD	veno-occlusive disease
vol	volume
VOR	vestibulo-ocular reflex
VORB	verbal order read back
VP	venipuncture; ventriculoperitoneal; venous pressure
VPAP	variable positive airway pressure

VPB	ventricular premature beat
VPC	ventricular premature contraction
VPI	velopharyngeal insufficiency
VPS	ventriculoperitoneal shunt
V/Q ratio	ventilation to perfusion ratio
VR	valve replacement; vascular resistance; venous return
VRA	visual reinforcement audiometry
VRE	vancomycin-resistant Enterococcus
VRSA	vancomycin-resistant Staphylococcus aureus
VS	vesicular sound; vestibular schwannoma; vital signs
VSD	ventricular septal defect
VSR	ventricular septal rupture
VSS	vital signs stable
VT, V-tach	ventricular tachycardia
Vt, TV	tidal volume
VTE	venous thromboembolism
VTEC	verotoxin-producing Escherichia coli
VUR	vesicoureteral reflux
VV	varicose vein
v/v	volume per volume
VVC	vulvovaginal candidiasis
VW	ventral wall; vessel wall
VWD	ventral wall defect; von Willebrand disease
VWF	von Willebrand factor
VZIG	varicella zoster immune globulin
VZV	varicella zoster virus
W	watt

w/	with
WA	while awake
WAIS	Wechsler Adult Intelligence Scale
WAP	wandering atrial pacemaker
WAS	Wiskott-Aldrich syndrome
WASP	Wiskott-Aldrich syndrome protein
WAT	white adipose tissue
WB	weight bearing; western blot; whole blood
WBAT	weight bearing as tolerated
WBC	white blood cell; white blood count
WBI	whole bowel irrigation
WBR	whole body radiation
WD	well-developed
w/d	withdrawal
WDL	within defined limit
WD/WN	well-developed/well-nourished
WEE	Western equine encephalitis
w/f	with food
WFL	within functional limit
WG	Wegener's granulomatosis
WH	well-hydrated
WHO	World Health Organization
WI	wound infection; wound irrigation
w/i	within
WIA	wounded in action
WIC	Special Supplemental Nutrition Program for Women, Infants, and Children
wid	widow/widower
WISC	Wechsler Intelligence Scale for Children

wk	week
WKS	Wernicke-Korsakoff syndrome
WLE	wide local excision
WM	white matter
WMA	wall motion abnormality
WN	well-nourished
WNL	within normal limit
WNV	West Nile virus
WN/WD	well-nourished/well-developed
WO	weeks old; wide open; written order
w/o	without
WOB	work of breathing
WPD	warm, pink, dry
WPWS	Wolff-Parkinson-White syndrome
WS*	Waardenburg syndrome*; Werner syndrome*; West syndrome*; Williams syndrome*; Wolfram syndrome*
wt	weight
WTD	wet to dry
w/u	workup
w/v	weight per volume
w/w	weight per weight
x	multiply by; times
x10d, FXD	for 10 days
x/7	x number of days
x/12	x number of months
x/40	x number of weeks of pregnancy
x/52	x number of weeks
X&D	examination and diagnosis

XDP, XP	xeroderma pigmentosum
xfer, TRF	transfer
XL	extended release; extra large
XM	crossmatch
XMM	xeromammogram; xeromammography
XR	extended release; x-ray
XRT, RT, RTx	radiation therapy; radiotherapy
Y-BOCS	Yale-Brown Obsessive Compulsive Scale
YF	yellow fever
YLC	youngest living child
YO, y/o	years old
YOA	years of age
YOB	year of birth
YPLL	years of potential life lost
yr	year
YST	yolk sac tumor
YTD	year-to-date
Z	atomic number (Zahl)
ZD	zinc deficiency
Z-DNA	left-handed DNA
ZE	Zollinger-Ellison
ZES	Zollinger-Ellison syndrome
ZIFT	zygote intrafallopian transfer
ZMC	zygomaticomaxillary complex
Zn	zinc
ZPIC	Zone Program Integrity Contractor
Z-RNA	left-handed RNA
ZSB	zero stools since birth
ZSR	zeta sedimentation ratio